Dr. Cass Ingram's

Natural Cures *for* Killer Germs

Knowledge House
Buffalo Grove, Illinois

Printed in the United States of America
First Edition

Disclaimer: This book is not intended as a substitute for medical diagnosis or
treatment. Anyone who has a serious disease should consult a physician before
initiating any change in treatment or before beginning any new treatment.

Printed on recycled paper

ISBN: 1-931078-10-6

For ordering information call (800) 243-5242 or send an email to droregano@aol.com.
For overseas orders call 1-847-473-4700 or order from vivanatura.nl.
For an informative Web site see www. oreganol.com

Table of Contents

Introduction

There is a cover-up in the United States. The powers-that-be claim all is under control. However, this is far from the case.

There are serious epidemics occurring in this country and modern medicine is impotent in stopping them. These epidemics could spread rapidly—overnight—developing into uncontrollable contagion. The entire world could be afflicted with such a contagion. The latter is known as a pandemic. In contrast, an epidemic is a small scale type of contagion, which might affect a region, perhaps even a city or state. It could also affect an entire country. In contrast, a pandemic is global, affecting uncountable individuals. America is highly vulnerable. It cannot escape. This is a serious time, and it must be regarded seriously.

Regarding the risks for a pandemic in America, for most people there is a nonchalance. It is as if Americans feel immune to the kind of debacle that, for instance, regarding the SARS epidemic, has occurred in China, Hong Kong, and Toronto. Americans are far from immune, in fact, they are already suffering. Americans are constantly afflicted with infectious diseases that are virtual outright epidemics. AIDS, hepatitis C, genital herpes, mycoplasma, drug-resistant staph/strep,

Epstein-Barr, genital warts, leukemia viruses, and TB are just a few examples.

An overwhelming international epidemic, which strikes every region of this globe, is merely a matter of time. The fact is it will happen soon, certainly within the reader's lifetime. The exact onset is unknown. However, current global events lean towards its sudden arrival. It may happen this year or next year or perhaps five years from now. Yet, the fact is it is inevitable. Thus, why rely upon apathetic authorities, who couch words and who may, in fact, feel compelled to minimize or even disguise the risks? Rather, wouldn't it make sense to take responsibility, that is to prepare for this issue yourself?

Since it is inevitable, it only makes sense to prepare. Regarding an individual's personal protection what else is there? Medicine offers no hope. For instance, despite decades of research medically, there is no cure for AIDS. Cancer and heart disease are regarded as incurable. Here, tens of billions of dollars have been spent, all for naught. Arthritis, Alzheimer's disease, Parkinson's disease, ALS, multiple sclerosis, asthma, emphysema, Crohn's disease, diabetes, fibromyalgia, chronic fatigue syndrome, and migraine headaches, all are without cures. Thus, since the vast majority of diseases are medically incurable any proposed cure should be investigated. This is the sensible approach to take. Even so, substantiation should be sought. Does such a cure have a reasonable basis? Is there any science substantiating it? Does it make medical sense to apply it? Are there any contraindications?

Now is the time to prepare, that is before the pandemic strikes. In the midst of it there is no time. It could strike and kill without warning. Thus, where do people turn? The fact is there are cures available, but they are outside of orthodox medicine. Thus, a person must search on his/her own to discover the truth, never relying on the authorities. With the sudden arrival of a tornado or earthquake, there is little or no warning. If you wait, it will probably be too late.

It is merely a matter of time. You may be in the midst of it or may escape it. If you escape it, perhaps your children or grandchildren will be the victims. However, ultimately, it will strike, and it will kill by the thousands and perhaps millions.

Pandemics are already killing by the millions. The devastation in Africa is an excellent example. AIDS and/or AIDS-like syndromes are destroying that continent. The cause is unknown. In its vast history it has never before been swept by such a disease. Perhaps vaccinations play a role in such an epidemic. Perhaps malnutrition is the primary issue. Perhaps it is a combination of such factors. Thus, epidemics, in fact, a wide range of them are already here. Some are man-made and others are the products of nature. What's more, sudden death of an unfathomable degree is only a matter of time. Yet, such dire consequences are far from inevitable, that is if the individual takes the appropriate actions. The fact is by following the advice in this book premature death from an epidemic can be prevented, regardless of the circumstances.

In modern medicine diseases seem so unapproachable. A diagnosis seems so frightening. The disease itself becomes a source of fear. It develops a power of its own, while seeming impossible to conquer. Is it that the disease is given too much power? Maybe diseases are not so invincible after all.

Epidemics can be conquered. What's more, the answers are found in nature.

During my medical training I was constantly exposed to the standard approach: no cure except drugs or surgery. Or, simply "There is no cure". I didn't believe it. I believed there must be a way to cure disease. It was the Prophet Muhammad who said, "For each disease God has created its cure." The Prophet gives hope; modern medicine removes it. Yet, in each case the exact cure had to be researched, perhaps tested. The secret is to find the exact cure a given disease requires.

Through some 20 years of practice I have discovered an inordinate amount of cures for diseases. Each cure is based upon the physiology of a given disease. Eventually, I found many cures and proved that many of the so-called incurable diseases could be completely reversed. M.J. is an excellent example. She had an "incurable" case of Epstein-Barr Syndrome. In this syndrome a herpes-like virus attacks the liver, ultimately destroying it. No one had been able to help her, even in the nutritional and herbal fields. I reasoned that the virus could be destroyed but that the treatment must be aggressive. Knowing that raw onions are highly antiviral plus they are safe for liver tissue, in fact, they help heal damaged liver tissue, I recommended a rather dramatic cure: raw onion juice. She was to juice yellow onions, which are particularly antiseptic. Parsley juice was added to minimize the odor. Next she was to buy the most potent radishes she could find, preferably black Russian or diakon. Then, she was to drink two cups of such a concoction daily. With some trepidation, although, in fact, she was open-minded about it, she did so. Within a week she felt remarkably better. Within a month the liver enzymes returned to normal. Mary Jane was cured, the condition never to return.

It is realized that this is an extreme case, that is the therapy was extreme. Yet, this patient's life was at risk. Due to her horrifying symptoms she was miserable. Her marriage was strained. A bit of discomfort, an awful taste was all that was required for a cure.

Nature has exceptionally potent cures. No government or vested interest can deny this. Nor can any such agency truly regulate it. The fact is major corporations are constantly searching for natural cures, largely to develop patentable medicines.

There are dozens of books about epidemics. This is the only one that describes cures. The fact is it is the only one which explains precisely what to do, that is when killer epidemics strike.

When global infections strike, the individual must be fully aware of what to do. There is no margin of error; there is no time for research. The individual must be capable of reacting immediately, that is to save his own self and any loved ones and then, if energy and resources permit, friends and associates as well as the needy stranger.

Epidemics already kill vastly. In fact, each year millions die from them. AIDS, hepatitis C, malaria, diarrheal diseases, and tuberculosis are continuous pandemics. The death toll yearly from these infections is in the tens of millions. Yet, all are curable. Perhaps the cure is known but not popularized. Or, perhaps it is yet to be found. Even so, for epidemics, as well as the vast majority of common diseases, there will never be a medical cure. Only nature can cure. This is where the cures will be found. Thus, while medicine is impotent in stemming the tide of infectious diseases, nature offers answers. The fact is nature, that is almighty God, provides a wide range of cures.

Medical professionals resist the use of the word cure for any substance, that is other than what is "recognized". Yet, the medical system uses natural substances, claiming them curative, for instance, the anti-cancer drug Taxol. Incredibly, for heart disease doctors often prescribe wine, obviously a natural substance. They have little basis to claim it as a cure, that is since alcohol is directly toxic to the arteries and heart muscle, yet they recommend it freely. Despite this they find it implausible that simple herbs or foods can cure. Aspirin and digitalis were originally herbal. There is no denying their pharmacological actions. The fact is digitalis, which is entirely herbal (or, rather, an extract of an herb), is "curative" for certain heart disorders. Thus, it is to be expected that natural medicines can cure, even rather simplistic ones such as garlic, onion, and wild oregano. Indeed, for centuries such medicines have been relied upon to cure and prevent disease. The only difference today is that there exists a financial lobby, which resists, in fact, fully fights, their use. There was no such lobby in antiquity. That is why ancient herbal books specifically and unabashedly mention the curative properties of various herbs, spices, and foods. These books outright claim natural substances, including various herbs, as cures. If they were curative previously, certainly, they would be curative today. The fact is a plethora of scientific studies document the potent curative properties of natural compounds. If the proper form and quality are used, natural substances are potent medicines. They have actions equally as powerful as many drugs and in many instances far more powerful.

High quality natural substances must be made available to all people. There should be no effort to restrict their availability. Herbal medicines are extensively targeted. A vast assault is levelled against them, much of it unjustified. Propaganda is unleashed, aimed to crush the herbal movement. True, certain herbs possess toxicity, for instance, ephedra. Yet, such toxicity is rare, in fact, incomparably so, versus drugs. Ephedra kills rarely; drugs kill commonly. What's more, ephedra itself is more drug-like rather than herbal. In contrast, the herbal form, ma haung, is relatively safe and has not been associated with sudden death.

Herbs are made from a source other than humans, that is the unfathomable and divine. In contrast, drugs are human concoctions or perhaps derivatives of nature. Natural medicines are highly safe, rarely causing organ toxicity and even more rarely causing death. In contrast, millions of Americans suffer organ toxicity from drugs. The fact is the regular use of virtually any drug will result in tissue damage. The uncontrolled use of such drugs results in uncountable cases of organ failure and death. This is the difference between the divinely created medicines and the man-made. Who can now argue against the value of herbal or natural medicines? The fact is anyone who restricts them, while fully aware of their value, is an accessory to human despair, injury, disease, and death.

A variety of natural compounds are drug-like. In other words, they exert significant actions upon human function. These actions may be readily proven through scientific studies. These are the types of agents—substances with a high degree of potency—which are recommended in this book. They are agents which, in fact, assist the body in the healing process, even outright reversing disease. They do so without causing significant harm. Nor do they cause serious side effects. What's more, they offer a potency and utility unavailable through modern medical drugs. This book only deals with natural medicines, which have been proven effective by laboratory and clinical studies as well as everyday human use.

Human beings have corrupted the Earth. They have also corrupted the food supply as well as water. Human meddling, as well as greed, has resulted in uncountable epidemics. Human beings are dying on a daily basis, and it is largely preventable. It is as if human life has little if any value. The deaths are mere statistics. The cause is largely ignored. Yet, the issue is what if it is personal: if it is your loved one—spouse, child, mother, father, or friend? What if such a person is the victim? Rather, what if the reader is, in fact, the victim? Now the reality of this debacle is made evident: all humans are victims of preventable diseases, if the individual only knew. This book describes the underlying causes of epidemics, human or natural, plus what can be done to prevent them. Yet, it provides another realm of information unavailable from modern medicine: what can be done to cure them.

Chapter 1
Under Siege

In the United States infectious diseases are running rampant. Most people are unaware of the risks. The plagues are already here, systematically eroding human health. In general, the medical profession refuses to admit to the severity of such public health challenges. Consumed by apathy and indifference it remains static, failing to take any significant action. This is largely because of its philosophy of "treat the symptoms" rather than treating the cause of disease. Even if action were taken, the medical system is hopelessly inadequate in its ability to respond, that is regarding pandemic germs. The fact is it fails to offer even a single cure. West Nile is killing and maiming Americans, plus animals, particularly birds and horses. What's more, SARS or SARS-like illnesses have killed dozens of Americans, although this information has been withheld. TB is resurging, even in the United States and Canada. Plus, intestinal parasitic infections are a fulminant epidemic, not just in the Third World, but right here in North America. Yet, despite this unrelenting assault not a single cure has been disseminated, nor any preventive measures. Thus, essentially, when epidemics strike, Americans are helpless. The government is impotent, offering no hope for emerging diseases. What's more, regarding natural cures there is little if any effort from the authorities. When a major pandemic breaks out, affecting tens of millions of Americans, there will be no means for the public to protect itself. The fact is people will be at the mercy of the medical system, which is woefully unprepared. Rather than offering cures hospitals and medical clinics will become a death zone. SARS is a disease primarily of hospitals. This is where the majority of people contract it. Thus, health care workers of all types are among the primary victims. Thus, the hospital is no place to be for a healthy or vulnerable person. Yet, in Hong Kong and China SARS has also stricken the general public, causing mass chaos.

In the late 1990s during international travels I made a first-ever observation. People who live vital and long lives had one thing in common. They regularly consume antiseptic herbs or foods in the diet. In other words, as a part of their native dietary habits they were unwittingly killing or warding off germs. By reducing the germ load within their bodies, and, thus, by warding off potentially life-threatening infections, they live longer. They didn't do it intentionally, it is just their way. In contrast to the American way of thinking they fail to consider that their habit will make them live longer or be free of disease. Often, they consume such germ-killing foods or beverages because they like the taste. Raw honey, vinegar, garlic, onions, sage, cilantro, radishes, turnips, hot-tasting greens, hot peppers, and oregano, these are consumed plentifully and regularly. Yet, so is yogurt, with its vast germ-fighting capacities. Fresh yogurt made from raw or even boiled milk is on the daily menu of many villagers. In the cities it is either fresh or pasteurized. In both cases it is loaded with healthy cultures, giving the intestines vital and disease-preventing quantities of healthy bacteria. Black tea, a mild antiseptic, is a staple, up to 10 cups daily, although, ostensibly, it is corrupted by the addition of prodigious amounts of sugar. Then, there are the glorious herbal teas, not the weak, devitalized, commercially available types, which have lost their aromatic essences, but, instead, the actual sprigs fresh from the mountains or the freshly ground herb. Such mountain-fresh teas are full of potent aromatics. It is the aromatics which provide germicidal actions. Without them the teas are ineffective as immune tonics. The fresh aroma and taste of aromatic compounds in the untarnished village teas: how completely different from the Western experience it is. It is a daily routine; hardly anyone misses a dose. Essentially, if you are a guest it is "forced" upon you.

The American diet is notoriously bland. Many Americans shy away from eating spicy fair. They claim they cannot tolerate it, that it upsets their digestion, and that their systems are too sensitive. They may even claim that spices damage their stomachs, perhaps causing actual illnesses, like heartburn and ulcers. The fact is rather than boosting immunity, much of the food in America depresses it. Americans are in a weakened state, in no condition for exposure to epidemic/pandemic germs. Thus, for millions of Americans spicy foods are vigorously avoided. As a result, the non-spice eaters are highly vulnerable to a variety of diseases, since spices are among the most potent sources of biological substances which protect the body from disease.

Again, consider the American diet, so rich in relatively bland foods such as white sugar, candies, cookies, cakes, pies, doughnuts, sweet rolls, bagels, bread, rolls, buns, cheese, well done meat, milk, potatoes, overdone vegetables, and cereal. It is easy to understand why Americans are vulnerable. With the exception of ethnic populations, who are, therefore, somewhat immunized, it is rarely spicy. None of the typical American foods offers even the slightest degree of antiseptic power.

Rather, such foods encourage the growth within our bodies of microbes. A teaspoon of white sugar is sufficient to halt the function of billions of white blood cells, while causing the growth of billions of yeasts. Imagine what happens if a person consumes it by the tablespoon daily. The fact is there are some Americans who consume as much as a cup of sugar daily as hidden or obvious calories. For instance, a single soda has some seven teaspoons of this deadly substance. A doughnut has up to ten teaspoons. Anyone who consumes large quantities is simultaneously feeding germs, which cause chronic immune suppression, as well as infections, especially by yeasts. The fact is a single teaspoon of refined sugar is sufficient to generate the growth of millions of yeasts and molds within the body. This explains the significant immunosuppressive actions of this substance. The fact is refined sugar is regarded by the body as a poison. Strictly avoid its consumption.

Kids are major sugar eaters. This extensive sugar ingestion greatly weakens their immune systems, making them vulnerable to microbial attack. Many children, due to their faulty diets, are microbial breweries, overpopulated by untold trillions of disease-causing germs. They are thus a sort of living microbial brewery, seeding infections to any near them. If a pandemic strikes, they will be exceptionally vulnerable. So will those who care for them. Thus, their diets must be radically improved. Otherwise, they may well die in vast numbers.

The purpose of this book is to stop pandemics. It gives dependable solutions. It provides solutions based upon facts: modern science. It is to create positive, that is effective, action. Ultimately, it is the means to save lives and prevent uncountable harm.

Germs can kill rapidly, far more rapidly than people are accustomed. If they develop a certain degree of virulence, they can kill before any therapy can be administered. This is what happened in 1918, when the pandemic virus mutated to a form which was capable of killing almost instantly, in some cases within 24 to 48 hours. The best defense is a powerful immune system. This is built through excellent diet as well as through avoiding toxic foods and beverages. What's more, the key is to know the power of natural cures, which specifically kill cold and flu viruses. This book provides such information in detail.

The Western world, despite its refinements and advances, is far from immune from pandemics. Infectious diseases of all types will strike here as easily as other less "fortunate" nations. As any review of history proves it is, in fact, the advanced civilizations which suffer "plague and pestilence." Even for the finest civilizations major pandemics always strike, usually unexpectedly. Often, it happens during a civilization's decline. This is when it is most vulnerable, when it is weak physically as well as spiritually. It is when its spirit is weakest when plagues strike fiercely. It happened in ancient Egypt, Greece, and Rome: all were devastated. All were crippled. All were ultimately crushed. What's more, it always struck unexpectedly. Yet, this is a different era. True, like the ancients American civilization is vulnerable. It is in decline. Seemingly, it is self-destructing. Its people are stressed and sick. Yet, while it is self-destructing, it inflicts untold damage upon all others. The same substances which have made its people direly ill are being foisted upon other nations: processed and adulterated food, genetically altered food, noxious drugs, and destructive vaccines. Thus, while America is direly ill, it is causing the entire human population to suffer, creating untold millions of victims globally.

The economic stresses are considerable, in fact, dire. People are so stressed out that they are making themselves sick. Human stress levels are far higher than anything known in ancient times. Yet, there exist today benefits unavailable to the ancients. There is a sophistication in modern society, as well as the information network, that could allow modern humans to defeat the pandemic. It will require a monumental effort, but it is possible, and that is what makes today's world unique in all history. Human beings can prepare and they can learn from history. Yet, learning is insufficient. It is necessary to take action based upon it. That is what makes us unique.

The modern era has heralded a reduction in the frequency of uncontrollable epidemics, that is the acute kind such as smallpox, typhus, yellow fever, cholera, and the flu. Yet, new threats have emerged, which are equally grave. AIDS, West Nile, Ebola, Cruetzfeldt-Jakob (i.e. the human version of mad cow), and SARS are perhaps more frightening than the previous killers.

The present era carries risks previously unknown. Simple measures, including the collection of garbage, the purification of water, the boiling of water, proper sewage disposal, and bathing, have reduced the incidence of disease astronomically. However, this is not the case with modern epidemics; they rampage throughout humanity despite such precautions. Here, there is no way to fully protect the people merely through public health measures. Chronic fatigue syndrome, fibromyalgia, Lyme, AIDS, West Nile, TB, hepatitis, and SARS ravage humanity, even in the most hygienic and sanitary countries. Obviously, there is no simplistic means for controlling such diseases. Only a highly aggressive approach aimed at strengthening immunity, as well as destroying germs, can succeed.

The tiniest monsters: stealth viruses

Viruses deplete the vitality from whatever they invade. They essentially subjugate the cells, draining them of all vitality, until they die. In essence, they are cellular hijackers, manipulating the genetic machinery of the cells to serve their destructive objectives. With stealth viruses, such as HIV, encephalitis viruses, and SARS, the body is overtaken before it even can mount a defense. Such viruses sneak into the cells, secretly invading them, then multiplying in uncountable numbers. All this occurs while they utterly evade immune defenses.

Normally, viruses cause an immune response. This is not the case with stealth viruses. The immune system is simply unable to detect them to the degree that it can mount a successful immune response. White blood cells respond by secreting chemicals, which provoke fever, a process which aids in killing viruses. They also produce antibodies, which bind to the viruses, speeding their destruction by white blood cells. Yet, this fails to occur during stealth virus infections. What's more, it is well known that there is no reliable medical treatment for viral infections. What are people to do in the event of a lethal pandemic?

When viruses enter the body, they attach to cells. Then, they begin their aggression. If they are prevented from attaching, they are defeated. However, once they attach, they readily invade. The body needs help in destroying them. That help comes from nature. It is the only hope humankind has for the prevention and cure of lethal modern infections.

It is humankind that has created modern monsters: tiny germs capable of killing and, more diabolically, utterly evading the immune system. These stealth germs are largely man-made, the products of so-called genetic engineering. Only synthetic drugs, as well as artificial genetic manipulations, could be responsible for such a disaster.

As late as the 1900s the cause of epidemic diseases was unknown. The study of microbes is a relatively new science, some 100 years old. Few cures have been popularized, that is except antibiotics. At one time synthetic phenol, that is carbolic acid, was extensively used. Made from coal tar, it was abandoned as a result of the introduction of antibiotics. Iodine was used, both internally and topically. Incredibly, despite research proving efficacy medicine has entirely failed to investigate natural antibiotics and antiseptics: there are tens of thousands of them. Rather, the entire focus has been on synthetic substances or natural compounds that have been extensively altered, all in the name of the creation of patentable medicines. This is despite the fact that antibiotics are highly limited in their use. With few exceptions antibiotics only kill bacteria. In contrast, antiseptics are naturally occurring germ killers, What's more, antiseptics are *anti-sepsis* meaning they kill the full range of germs, that is bacteria, fungi, molds, viruses, and parasites. Drugs are incapable of killing viruses. Despite their apparent potency and lifesaving reputation antibiotics have utterly failed to control or cure disease. The fact is their persistent use causes certain diseases, notably mutant bacterial conditions such as drug-resistant staph, drug-resistant strep, and pseudomembranous enterocolitis. In fact, antibiotics today cause a greater number of diseases than they cure. For instance, an entire disease category, known as candidiasis, is largely due to antibiotic therapy. This disease afflicts tens of millions of Americans, including millions of children, who developed it primarily as a result of antibiotic use.

Medicine claims to have conquered numerous diseases. This is far from true. People are sick today more so than ever before, and this is largely as a consequence of modern medicine. As well, the vast intake of processed foods also plays a primary role. Infections are increasingly a cause of death; they are far from conquered. With perhaps the exception of smallpox all major infections continue to ravage humanity.

In North America there are a number of mysterious pockets where infectious diseases still devastate the masses. People in such regions are often chronically ill, but have no clue regarding the cause. There germs are infective and destructive, damaging the tissues. Doctors are unaware of the cause and incapable of providing effective treatment. A large percentage of these infections are caused by viruses, although fungi also play a prominent, if not equivalent, role.

"They are tiny" says Madeline Drexler in her book, *Secret Agents*, so small that "tens of millions can fit on a mere pin head." Outside of a living being viruses are lifeless, rather, dormant. They become infective only after they invade a cell. They do so through pure stealth. The fact is viruses are like secret agents. They penetrate a region undetected. They are specifically designed to penetrate and gain entrance to the cell, in fact even the cell nucleus. They maintain a special structure which evades the immune response through stealth. Thus, they evade and/or neutralize the cellular defenses. Only then can they reproduce. Only then can they infect human tissues.

There are several approaches to preventing their invasion. One is to block their invasion through improving the strength of the cells. In other words, if the outer coatings of the cells are in top condition, the viruses are less able to invade. This is achieved through proper nutrition. The ability of the immune system to recognize and destroy such invaders may also be enhanced. Proper nutrition helps here as well. Having a strong, nutritionally fit body is one of the best ways to resist pandemic germs. Yet, this is no guarantee. For instance, in the 1918 flu perfectly healthy individuals were killed. Even so, a nutritionally solid diet plus a supplement program is crucial as insurance against global killers.

The role of nutrition in the resistance against disease is indisputable. The health crisis in Africa is an excellent example. Here, people are the most malnourished in the world. Africans also have the world's highest death rate from AIDS and other global killers.

There is no relief from emerging infections. Seemingly, every day a new outbreak occurs. The medical system is fully unprepared for such outbreaks. Plus, it has no ability to cure any such diseases. Rather, modern medicine has created a vast number of debilitating infections and is even responsible for causing deaths. Uncountable numbers of Americans die every year as a consequence of the toxicity of antibiotics and cortisone, both of which create bizarre mutant germs. The germs created by such drugs ultimately kill the patients. Radiation therapy also causes germs to mutate, leading to disease, disability, and death. Vaccines also kill, maim, and debilitate. In contrast, natural herbal antiseptics, particularly oil of wild oregano from the edible spice, oil of cinnamon, oil of clove, and similar substances, never cause deaths. Even minor injuries due to such substances are relatively unknown. What a contrast it is: thousands of deaths yearly from drugs versus no deaths from food-based medicines.

Killer plagues are already afflicting Americans. People are dying unnecessarily. Deaths are occurring in all age categories, even children and teenagers. This depletes the fabric of civilization; people are killed before their time. The fact is the modern plagues kill many people in the primes of their lives. It is truly a dire crisis, and the consequence is the erosion of the strength of civilization. People are already dying prematurely from AIDS, mutant hospital germs, Lyme, tuberculosis, and West Nile. The medical system is overwhelmed by this crisis. It is unable to cope even with a single major epidemic. When the next pandemic strikes, how could it handle that?

SARS is one such pandemic, although the incidence is in significant decline. This is the abbreviation for severe acute respiratory syndrome. No one is certain who coined this name. It would more properly be named a pandemic flu-like virus. SARS is a kind of catch-all diagnosis. Certainly, in 2003 the patients who died in Kaiser Permanante had severe acute respiratory syndrome, in other words, SARS. Based upon the symptoms they exhibited there is no other conclusion.

Certain people are highly vulnerable to SARS. People who are over 60 are perhaps most vulnerable, especially those who have received adult vaccines, particularly the flu vaccine. In fact, vaccine administration is a major risk for developing SARS, especially its life-threatening form. This may account for the high vulnerability for SARS among hospital workers. With the exception of the military they are the most extensively vaccinated of all people. Other individuals with a high vulnerability for developing a potentially fatal type of SARS include people taking multiple drugs, those on anti-inflammatory medications, especially the so-called NSAIAs, anyone who regularly takes cortisone, and chemotherapy/radiation patients. The anti-inflammatory drugs are particularly vile. They directly inhibit the immune response, greatly increasing the risks for SARS or SARS-like infections.

Mold or fungal infection is another significant risk factor. Molds and various fungi, including yeasts, readily infect the body. There is an epidemic of infections of people by these organisms. Global warming and an increase in flooding are major contributors to the heightened exposure to mold. Of the various types of fungi molds are perhaps the most insidious. There is a virtual pandemic of mold infections in many regions of North America. Molds usually enter the body through inhalation, although both molds and their toxins may also be ingested. Ultimately, the molds enter the body, that is the blood and/or organs, where they multiply, causing infection.

A vast number of molds are now known to infect the body. They may invade virtually any organ and readily infect both the digestive tract and bloodstream. These molds include aspergillus, penicillium, stachybotrus, cladosporidium, and fusarium. Microbiologists are finding various molds in the bloodstreams of relatively normal people. However, the counts of these molds are highest in people who are chronically ill. Diseases associated with large amount of molds in the blood include chronic fatigue syndrome, polymyositis, fibromyalgia, arthritis, lupus, migraine headaches, bronchitis, sarcoidosis, asthma, emphysema, tuberculosis, and chronic sinusitis.

Once these molds become established in the body they greatly depress the immune system. Molds produce mycotoxins, which exert highly negative effects upon the immune system. The fact is mycotoxins are among the most potent immunosuppressive substances known. Matossian, in her book, *Poisons of the Past: Mold Epidemics and History*, correlates exposure to mycotoxins as a primary cause of catastrophic plagues. The various major pandemics of history, the types which have led to the decline or collapse of civilizations, are apparently due in part to mold and, therefore, mycotoxin poisoning. The molds and mycotoxins poisoned the people, largely as a result of the ingestion of wet/contaminated grain, damaging and depressing the immune systems of the masses. Their immune systems thereby weakened, the masses became highly vulnerable to the spread of germs, resulting in uncontrollable plagues.

Mycotoxins essentially neutralize the immune system. They also disrupt the hormone system and are particularly toxic to the reproductive system. This was demonstrated by a recent poisoning in animals. In Iowa both cows and pigs are becoming infertile from eating corn. The corn is genetically engineered. This engineering weakens the corn's immune system, making it highly vulnerable to mold infection. The engineered corn, which was fed to the animals, was found to be infected with fusarium fungus. Apparently, the mycotoxins from this fungus had fully contaminated the corn. When the toxin-contaminated corn was eaten, it completely disrupted the reproductive systems of the pigs and cows, rendering them infertile. Interestingly, when one of the farmers switched back to non-genetically engineered corn, the reproductive problems disappeared. Thus, not only were the fungal toxins causing the sickness but, apparently, some unknown contaminant(s) in the genetically engineered corn was also poisoning these animals. The fact is the meat of such animals must also be poisoned, which is a strong reason to avoid commercial meats. The option is to eat organically- or naturally-raised meats.

Corn, whether organic, genetically engineered, or 'regular', is notoriously contaminated with mold. This is largely a result of farming practices. If the corn is stored in silos, mold may readily grow upon it. If it is air dried and then properly packaged, mold will not grow. For mold to grow moisture plus darkness is required. Plus, mold readily grows on sugar. Thus, any food which is relatively high in it will support mold growth. Of all vegetables corn is highest in sugar. Fruit also readily sustains mold growth, the high sugar fruits being most vulnerable. Fruits highest in sugar include grapes, apples, pears, raisins, dates, figs (dried), and pears. Low sugar fruits include grapefruit, lemons, limes, strawberries, papaya, kiwi, and melons.

Mold may readily grow on virtually any food, that is except meat, eggs, and milk. For instance, nuts and seeds may contain high mold levels. Certain foods are relatively resistant to mold growth, for instance, hot spices such as mustard, cumin, sage, cayenne, garlic, oregano, bay leaf, and thyme. Yet, incredibly, both onions and garlic may sustain mold growth.

Besides corn various grains are major sources of mold. The grains which are most vulnerable include wheat and rye. For those who are mold sensitive avoidance of corn, wheat, and rye may be necessary.

Raw nuts and seeds may also be contaminated. To neutralize mycotoxins raw nuts and seeds may be gently roasted for a few minutes on low heat (i.e. 150 to 200 degrees). Wild or brown rice may be eaten as a starch source instead of commercial grains. To reduce exposure to mold eat only low sugar fruit such as grapefruit, kiwi (hard), watermelon, cassava, lemons, limes, blueberries, and fresh strawberries.

Mold contamination can be reduced through the use of spice extracts. Germ-a-Clenz multiple spice extract spray is ideal for this purpose. Simply spray on the outside of any suspect fruit and wipe. Or, spray directly into fruit and simply leave. The latter approach is ideal for strawberries, raspberries, blueberries, currants, blackberries, raisins, figs, dates, and similar soft or watery fruit. It may also be used to decontaminate fruit with hard outer surfaces. For instance, cantaloupe is an ideal fruit for the mold sensitive person, since it is low in sugar. However, it tends to develop mold infections on the surface. This is where Germ-a-Clenz is ideal. Simply spray on the cantaloupe and allow to sit. Rinse or leave to dry. Then, after an hour or two cut and serve. Watermelon may also be contaminated, since they rest directly upon the ground. Germ-a-Clenz readily cleans dirt off the rind, while killing mold. Simply spray and wipe off or allow it to remain and penetrate the fruit. For the mold sensitive Germ-a-Clenz is a boon. Through using it a greater variety of fruit will be tolerated.

Parasites are yet another issue with fresh fruit. Here, a spice oil-based spray can be highly protective. This is because spice oils destroy both parasites and their cysts. A wide range of parasites can be contracted from fresh fruit, including amoebas, the cause of dysentery, cryptosporidium, cyclospora, liver flukes, giardia, and roundworms. The point is to kill the parasites where they are most vulnerable: outside the body. Once they are ingested, they can often evade the killing actions of medicines by hiding deep in tissues or by invading cells, where they are relatively protected. This can fully be prevented by using a spice oil spray on all fresh produce, both fruits and vegetables. It may even be used in restaurants. Simply spray any uncooked food before eating. It adds a pleasant taste, while sterilizing the food.

With parasitic infections prevention is the key. This is where Germ-a-Clenz is invaluable. There is nothing more miserable than a severe parasitic infection from contaminated food or water. The diarrhea, cramps, pain, and fever are intolerable. Yet, it all could be prevented, that is with proper hygiene and the strategic use of spice oil sprays.

Germ-a-Clenz is instrumental in halting pandemics, whether due to viruses, bacteria, parasites, and/or molds. This is because it attacks the true cause of many pandemics: environmental germs. By attacking and destroying germs in the environment, the epidemic or pandemic is halted before it can strike. In other words, the germs are killed before they can harm or kill you. This is the immeasurable benefit of such a cleanser. It kills the germs which commonly infect humans. They are germs which are rendered impotent through a proper hygienic approach. Thus, such a substance, along with spice oil extracts, prevents disease and saves lives.

Chapter 2
Danger Zones, Everywhere

The world is more dangerous now than ever before, that is from an infectious disease perspective. The dangers are obvious. Germs can kill quickly, without warning. They can maim in mere minutes. They can destroy cells and organs in fractions of a second. They can kill despite the best medicine.

Now the germs have mutated into direly aggressive forms. There is no guarantee that the immune system by itself can kill them. This means that all people are vulnerable to sudden illness, even sudden death.

Why are today's germs so destructive? It is the human race which is largely responsible for this debacle. Human beings have created the majority of these monsters. Modern science is the primary culprit, supported by business interests. The greed and lust for money has led to an international catastrophe. Consider, for instance, the mutant staph and strep, which cause flesh-eating diseases. Prior to the introduction of antibiotics and other immunosuppressive drugs, such as cortisone and antiinflammatory drugs, no such diseases existed. The antibiotics have been over-used, especially in cattle. Doctors overprescribe them, even for conditions such as viral infections, for which they are worthless. What's more, they usually fail to warn the patients of the consequences: the creation of mutant-germs. These mutants are biological monsters, capable of causing widespread damage, even maiming and/or killing within minutes. Now the human race must create the solution or risk extinction.

Truly, microbes could destroy the human race. Certainly, as proven by the recent SARS and bird flu pandemics they are capable of disrupting humanity, damaging the medical, as well as financial, infrastructure of entire cities, in fact, countries. China, formerly a bastion of financial success, is on the verge of bankruptcy. Hong Kong is tottering dangerously close to financial collapse, as is Taiwan. Yet, how could it be? A mere microscopic cell, capable of bankrupting entire nations? Yet, this is precisely what is happening. Unless governments provide solutions to the microbial challenge, they will become bankrupt, medically and financially. Yet, governments will likely never solve this. This is because they are infiltrated with special interest groups. Such groups have no interest in the powers of nature. The fact is nature is impossible to patent. Anyone can recommend onion extract, raw honey, or oil of oregano. Anyone could sell it. Governments are controlled by big money interests. Regarding natural cures, it is this vested interest which interferes with freedom of expression. Certainly, it is far from any concern of danger or merely because such substances are "unregulated". The latter could easily be rectified, that is without draconian measures. What's more, natural cures threaten major financial interests. If people remain in perfect health, many companies would go out of business. Thus, efforts will be made to denigrate, in fact, obstruct, natural cures. In fact, in the United States, as well as Canada, there is a major effort to restrict access to such cures. This has already been achieved in Europe. The effort is intense to do so here.

Books give information about the scope of epidemics or pandemics. They describe the crisis facing humanity. They reveal the agony and despair—the death, destruction, and devastation. Yet, none can give answers. That is the difference between other books and this book. Here, definite cures are described, which reverse virtually all plagues.

There is no need to succumb to fatalism. Any infection may be cured. There may be no medical cure. Yet, nature offers potent medicines, which orthodox physicians may be unfamiliar with. The fact that the medical system has failed to do so is no indication of the possibilities. Consider acupuncture. It certainly eases pain, some studies showing that it works as well as chemical anesthetics.

Modern medicine often takes the exact opposite approach of the truth. For instance, in infants modern medicine has always promoted stomach sleeping. Yet, it has recently been proven that such an approach, in fact, causes deaths: from SIDS. By laying an infant on the stomach the weight against the stomach and esophagus causes regurgitation. The fluids fall back into the lungs, causing suffocation. This still occurs and it would be nearly completely rectified by back or side sleeping. In the case of sleeping position medicine faltered, commanding precisely the opposite from nature. God commands one method and medicine demands another: God is right, medical arrogance is wrong. The fact is due to this on-the-stomach mandate tens of thousands of babies died: an atrocious consequence. There are even mothers who have been falsely imprisoned, suspected of murdering their babies and the entire cause was stomach sleeping. This is despite the fact that stomach sleeping was prohibited far prior: in the seventh century by the Prophet Muhammad. Again, the point is if modern medicine fails to endorse an approach, that is of no consequence. Rather, the approach of modern medicine is biased, that is it pursues only that which supports its position—its medical monopoly—rather than that which is of value to the masses.

This is far from an attack against the medical community. It is merely the facts as they now exist. When emerging diseases strike—when vast illnesses overwhelm society—medicine will be impotent. It simply fails to produce any cure. That has been its history. There will be no change in this trend. What's more, those who rely exclusively on the medical system will be at risk for extermination. Those who doubt this system and prepare for their own battle will have the best chance for survival. They are the people who will likely survive the diabolical diseases of the future, in fact, of the present. This is because they will be armed with the answers. These are answers found exclusively in nature. Drugs cause a greater degree of disease than any cure. Thus, there is only nature, which is left to rely upon.

Nature is the source of all existing cures. Drugs originated in natural compounds, for instance, aspirin from white willow bark and digitalis from the herb foxglove. These drugs are still among the most commonly used today. Yet, they are altered and, thus, cannot be compared to their parent, that is natural, compounds. Drugs possess extensive toxicity. Natural compounds are rarely toxic. Drugs are a major cause of sudden death. A report in *JAMA* places the deaths in the United States from drugs, which are properly prescribed, at some 110,000 per year. In contrast, with the exception of ephedra, which is largely synthetic (that is purified), deaths from herbal medicines are nil. Even with ephedra compared to the number of people using it the death rate is essentially non-existent.

This fact should be given serious consideration. Can anyone prove considerable deaths in the United States from pure herbs or even potent herbal extracts? If there is skepticism, then list such deaths? Essentially, there are none. Yet, in North America alone the deaths from drugs may be as high as 350,000 per year, perhaps higher. This is because such deaths occur in a variety of ways. There are the aforementioned deaths from properly prescribed drugs. Yet, how many deaths occur from those which are improperly prescribed? Hospitals are the primary sites which record drug-induced deaths. How many other deaths occur, for instance, in outpatients, which are never reported or outright covered up? What's more, antibiotics, the most commonly prescribed of all drugs, cause their own types of deaths. These are deaths from monster germs, the so-called drug-resistant mutants. These mutant germs abound within hospitals, clinics, and doctors offices. People readily develop infections by such germs during hospitalization as well as during invasive treatments. Even the mere suturing of a wound can lead to a life-threatening infection. Again, *JAMA* claims the deaths are incredibly high: some 250,000 per year from medically induced sepsis, that is blood poisoning, alone. Thus, the admitted deaths are some 360,000. It is reasonable to estimate the remaining deaths, including deaths of patients who receive their drugs as samples or from pharmacies, at an additional 100,000, which is conservative. This places the total lives lost at 460,000. In contrast, yearly deaths from heart disease are over 700,000, while deaths from cancer are approximately 900,000. Thus, doctor- and hospital-induced deaths, rather, pharmaceutical house-induced deaths, are the third leading cause of fatality in the United States. This is a kind of murder. People place their trust in the drugs, perhaps failing to realize that such agents can kill. Yet, such a fraud persists without scrutiny or prosecution.

This is far from an attack upon the pharmaceutical houses. It is merely to set the record straight. Herbs are, essentially, non-toxic. Drugs are fulminant poisons. The major danger to the human race is drug therapy, not herbal medicine. Drugs must be more carefully regulated. Herbs, which also must be regulated, that is for quality and toxicity, are a lesser issue. True, if certain herbs do cause toxicity, this must be known. The public must be made fully aware of it. Such herbs should be taken with caution, if at all. Yet, herbs which are truly toxic are rare. Even with these death is virtually unknown. Over a 50 year period in the United States total deaths from herbal medicines are less than 100, while the total from pharmaceutical drugs numbers in the millions. It was during the 1950s that the pharmaceutical cartel became fully established. The total deaths for pharmaceutical drugs may be revealing. Since the 1950s a reasonable estimate for drug-induced deaths is approximately 2 million. This is based upon an average of some 50,000 deaths per year, which, surely, is conservative. Remember, the total deaths from pharmaceutical agents in a single year alone has been estimated at 300,000. 1.5 million versus 100: is there any comparison? The fact is even the figure of 100 is high, that is in terms of fully natural herbs. In other words, the deaths from the intake of edible herbs and spices such as garlic, onion, sage, cumin, cinnamon, cloves, and turmeric is significantly less if any. Regarding the latter not a single case has been recorded. Thus, the documented cases of deaths due to edible herbs and/or spices are few, especially with those which are food-like. Regarding food-like substances serious illness or death amounts to a few utterly rare allergic reactions. True, certain herbs are toxic. Examples include pennyroyal, chapparel, and artemesia. Yet, again, death due to such herbs is very rare.

Certain natural medicines are fully safe and can be taken with impunity. Such natural medicines are the focus of this book. In the years 2000 through 2003 there are no deaths on record from the ingestion of pure edible herbs, foods, or spices such as garlic, onion, oregano, cumin, sage, rosemary, turmeric, dandelion, coriander, and ginger. Rather, as a result of their intake lives have been saved. All the aforementioned herbs are medicinal. Herbs are natural drugs, and thus are quite capable of curing disease, while rarely if ever killing anyone. In contrast, synthetic drugs, which are incapable of curing disease, readily kill. The two cannot be compared. What's more, the choice, that is regarding which should be pursued, is obvious. While there are attempts to 'regulate' herbs, even restrict their availability, little if anything is being done to remove killer drugs from the market, including acetaminophen and aspirin. Such drugs are responsible for thousands of deaths yearly plus untold thousands of cases of irreversible poisoning. Nothing is done to curb or restrict their use. This is a travesty against humanity. Thus, in the United States regarding human health and safety financial interests rule, not the needs of humanity.

There are other reasons for the danger: suppression of the immune system. The immune system is a delicate 'organism'; noxious substances readily disrupt it. In particular, drugs quickly disable it. Drugs which aggressively damage the immune system include cortisone, non-steroidal antiinflammatory agents, antibiotics, methotrexate, chemotherapeutic agents, estrogen-based drugs, Dilantin, cholesterol-lowering agents, anti-rejection drugs, penicillamine, and birth control pills. In particular, cortisone, as well as prednisone and cortisone-based creams or inhalers, are of concern. These drugs rapidly suppress immunity, and if they are taken regularly for prolonged periods, irreversible immune damage occurs. Usually, the use of such agents is unnecessary; natural medicines can be applied. The medical profession uses cortisone to an excess, nearly always without sound clinical justification. In medicine today cortisone has become a generic therapy; that is when all else fails, it is prescribed or injected. This vague, unscientific approach causes great damage, even deaths, all of which is needless. In the Western world the inappropriate use or overuse of cortisone is a primary cause of disability and disease. Inhalers for asthmatics are a good example. Some researchers have documented a significant increase in deaths for asthmatics who use such inhalers versus those who don't. In other words, such cortisone-based inhalers, in fact, worsen the asthma, even causing deaths.

Every year thousands of asthmatics die as a result of these drugs. Incredibly, the very therapy which is prescribed increases the disability, sickness, hospitalization, and death rate in the vulnerable, suffering asthmatic. Such individuals would be better off if they simply avoided all medication. For instance, a study reported in *Family Practice News* documents as a result of steroid-based inhalers death rates have risen over 30%. In other words, asthmatics who failed to use the inhaler fared better than users. Doctors emphasize the use of inhalers for asthma. Yet, nutritional physicians achieve similar results, that is in the reduction of bronchospasm, with vitamin C, magnesium, and pantothenic acid—without increasing the death rate. This demonstrates why it is so dangerous to exclusively rely upon the medical system.

Antibiotics are also potentially noxious. A number of studies have demonstrated that such drugs suppress the immune system. Certain antibiotics, for instance, aminoglycosides, poison the bone marrow. In particular, chloramphenicol can cause irreversible bone marrow failure. Erythromycin can permanently destroy the liver. Tetracyclines can induce autoimmune diseases. Incredibly, these are mere antibiotics, which people take relatively freely.

In the majority of diseases it is more dangerous to receive orthodox treatment than to neglect it. This is represented by a well known observation made in the 1970s. In New York City when doctors went on strike for six months a noticeable decline occurred in the death rate. In other words, the lack of meddling with people's bodies through unnecessary surgeries and medications saved lives, even by six months. This is an incredible statistic. Yet, it fully illustrates the immense dangers of modern medicine, which is based upon the dictates of the drug and surgical cartels. "Protect financial interests at all costs" is the motto of such industries, even the cost of human lives.

Yet, while natural medicines are safer than drugs discretion must be taken here as well. Certain natural substances, for instance, aflatoxin, which contaminates corn and grain, are highly toxic. Even certain foods may upset chemistry, for instance, through food allergy reactions. If a person is allergic to a certain food, eating it can cause a wide range of symptoms: even illness or death. Common foods, such as wheat, corn, peanuts, and soy, can be highly disruptive to the system, weakening a person's resistance to disease. The heavy intake of commercial soy has been linked to brain and liver damage, as well as sexual disfunction in males, while wheat may cause destruction of the stomach and intestinal lining. Even water can be fatal, that is if it is drunk to an excess.

There is a science to natural medicine. A sensible approach is to evaluate each person's vulnerabilities and needs. Then, an individualized program may be designed to correct any imbalances, excesses, and deficiencies. This ideal is difficult to achieve. Only a trained nutritionally oriented practitioner can do so. However, people can help the self towards health improvement, since certain general rules apply. People who are chronically ill usually suffer from food allergies. What's more, they usually have numerous nutritional deficiencies. If the dietary and nutritional components are corrected, the health is improved. For this purpose a specialized system available only on the internet may prove invaluable. Called Nutritiontest.com here an individual can fully determine his/her precise nutritional and dietary needs.

People who are ill are often toxic. They suffer from a state of toxin overload in their internal organs and blood. In particular, the liver, kidneys, bloodstream, spleen, and intestines are readily poisoned. These organs can be cleansed through herbal detoxification or via various purges. What's more, certain foods are universal allergens. Soy, corn, peanuts, and wheat may be avoided: most people will notice improved overall health simply by removing them. Other foods highly likely to disrupt body chemistry include chocolate, red wine, certain cheeses, cow's milk, and citrus. Commercial food additives are also highly disruptive. The list includes sulfites, nitrates, MSG, food dyes, and aspartame. If the aforementioned foods and additives are avoided, in most individuals there will be significant health improvement. This is a start in a positive direction. A nutritionally oriented practitioner can refine this further. Or, an individual can determine his/her own dietary and nutritional status conveniently through Nutritiontest.com. The Nutritiontest system is highly accurate and, thus, it produces superior results than even that which is normally gained by seeing a nutritionist or even a doctor. One person took the tests and found out she was deficient in selenium. She followed the advice, that is her appropriate intake of selenium supplements plus selenium-rich foods. As a result, her illness—psoriasis—disappeared.

Danger zones, everywhere

There are danger zones everywhere. There is no question that they exist. A person is feeling well then, suddenly, becomes violently ill. Such a degree of danger is truly modern. Yes, there were epidemics of old. However, today there are modern diseases, which strike suddenly and are equally as fatal as the more ancient types. Yet, still, somehow, it is different. These modern germs are mutations, and they are exceptionally vicious. Today, it is supposed to be safe, certainly, safer than the previous centuries. However, in many respects it is even more dangerous than ever before. Incredibly, they are found in any region, particularly outside of the home: restaurants, picnics, theatres, airplanes, cruise ships, malls, hotels, sporting arenas, and more: anyplace where people congregate. Areas where food is handled are particularly treacherous. Closed spaces are danger zones, especially airplanes and cruise ships. People are compacted within these spaces. Thus, in these environments germs can spread readily. Hospitals are utter catastrophes. There, a pathogen can be contracted readily, merely by breathing the air.

The powers of Germ-a-Clenz: nature's air purifier

Spice oils, which are germicidal, can be converted into an effective spray. Such a spray, known as Germ-a-Clenz, purges the air of pathogens, while creating a natural immune-boosting odor. The fact is Germ-a-Clenz enlivens the senses, while killing germs. It also opens the sinuses, which synthetic air cleaners are incapable of achieving. Chemical germicides and deodorizers, in fact, depress immunity and may also cause allergic reactions. People are highly sensitive to synthetic chemicals, which, while possibly killing germs, also damage human cells. This is why Germ-a-Clenz is invaluable. It is completely non-toxic to human tissues. Plus, it destroys pathogens, which are responsible for pandemics. The majority of such infections spread through the air. Germ-a-Clenz interrupts this cycle. Thus, by purging the air of pathogens it interrupts the spread of dangerous germs. It does this because it neutralizes the germs before they can inflict damage. Thus, it helps stop pandemics before they can kill. When visiting anyone in a hospital, be sure to take it with you. Spray it into the air. Also, rub the hands with oil of wild oregano (Oreganol P73) before entering the hospital and while leaving. What's more, to safeguard the body take a few drops under the tongue before entering. Rub a few drops under the nose as protective aromatherapy.

The winter is a danger zone. With SARS, it could bring catastrophe. Respiratory infections are notoriously brutal during the winter. During the winter of 2003 a SARS-like syndrome began spreading in the United States, particularly on the West Coast. People were developing a kind of hemorrhagic flu, which is typical of this infection. SARS plus the flu may be more than the human race, as well as the medical infrastructure, can withstand. The coronavirus and similar animal-source viruses are hardy. They can withstand the extremes of heat and cold. Tests prove that the coronavirus which causes SARS can withstand freezing temperatures as low as -110 degrees Fahrenheit. This presents a potentially dire scenario: a massive outbreak of the virus in the winter, when there is no sunlight to sterilize the air. Thus, the virus, unimpeded, spreads readily in the winter air, entering buildings, where it is inhaled. It attacks the respiratory tract aggressively, lodging within cells. It begins reproducing immediately. A highly aggressive germ, eventually, it overwhelms the lungs' immune defenses. It attacks the lung cells, ultimately destroying them. This leads to bleeding, which occurs mainly in the lower parts of the lungs. The lungs turn into a kind of mushy tissue, appearing like raw liver. Then, bleeding develops in other organs, including the liver and spleen. The blood count suddenly plunges, and the blood pressure drops. Blood pours from every orifice. Rapidly, the individual succumbs and dies. Thus, SARS is truly a hemorrhagic fever, with features similar to Ebola.

Since the initial outbreak the SARS incidence has significantly declined. Yet, this virus could mutate into a highly virulent form, especially in the fall and winter. This is far from mere hype. Rather, it is a historical fact. The SARS virus is similar to the original 1918 flu virus. Like this earlier virus it causes a rapid decline in health, affecting a wide range of organ systems. Both the SARS virus and the 1918 germ killed by causing internal bleeding. In other words, both are hemorrhagic viruses. Thus, they attack any and all tissues at will. Both of these viruses spread via super-infectors, who are capable of infecting dozens of people. What's more, both were capable of destroying entire organ systems, including the lungs, heart, spleen, liver, and kidneys. The only guarantee for survival is to kill such viruses: directly within the human body.

In the winter the lungs are significantly compromised. Germs abound in indoor air. Colds and flu depress the immune system. This makes the individual vulnerable to even more aggressive germs such as the SARS virus. In a weakened state, a person who would normally fight it off could succumb. This could happen quickly, that is within a few hours. Or, it might happen over a longer period: a few highly miserable days or weeks.

Hemorrhagic viruses, such as the SARS and bird flu viruses, are potent killers. They must be attacked aggressively. The immune system by itself is often unable to defeat them. This is why spice extracts are so crucial. They represent the only natural substances which reliably destroy such germs. Spice extracts, in fact, destroy the coronavirus, that is the virus which causes SARS. A recent study performed at Microbiotest Labs found that a tiny amount of a commercially available product, Oregacyn P73, utterly destroyed all traces of this virus. The Oregacyn in a mere concentration of a tenth of a percent (.01) destroyed in tissue culture tens of millions of coronaviruses. Yet, it works in the human body as well. Dr. Naima Abdel-Ghany has shown that in humans suffering from hepatitis C spice extracts made from wild material, that is the Oreganol and Oregacyn, destroy hepatitis C viruses. In one individual blood levels of hepatitis C dropped from some 5 million per milliliter to only 450. That is a tremendous response.

The same response is expected even in pandemic infections, although massive doses may be necessary. This is because in fulminant infections untold billions, in fact, trillions, of viruses are within the body, attacking the individual. This is typical of sudden viral syndrome: a massively overwhelmed immune system, unable to cope with the multitudes of germs. This is the challenge of acute viral infections: destroying the viruses before they destroy you. Such an attack may require massive doses of combined therapy: Oreganol P73 under the tongue, a few drops even every few minutes plus, orally, the Oregacyn, a few capsules every hour. Oregacyn is ideal for another reason: it is hemostatic, meaning it halts bleeding. This is another reason Oregacyn saves lives.

When epidemics strike, there is no reason to panic or lose hope. Natural medicines, particularly wild spice extracts, effectively kill germs. Goldenseal, echinacea, elderberry, grapefruit seed extract, and colloidal silver are alternatives, however, they cannot be relied upon. Only spice extracts, such as Oreganol and Oregacyn, have been proven in clinical trials to destroy potentially fatal germs.

Epidemic germs can prove aggressive and can rapidly threaten lives. The key is to be aggressive with the therapy. Spice extracts will save lives, that is if the individual is persistent, that is if the person takes a sufficient quantity. For instance, in dire circumstances it may be necessary to take the Oreganol and Oregacyn every hour, even every few minutes. It is a matter of killing the virus, before it kills you.

Invisible but deadly

The word virus is commonly misused, especially by the media. Thus, this germ is the subject of a great deal of misinformation. A wide range of infections are described as viral infections, even though they are not. Viruses are the tiniest of microbes, although there may be smaller ones, which are unknown. Because of their size they are highly invasive. They are not alive. Thus, to survive they must invade living tissue. The term itself, which comes from the Latin word for poison, was originally used to describe contagion caused by a variety of germs.

Viruses cause specific types of infections. Incredibly, in newspapers infections caused by bacteria are often described as viral. This demonstrates the degree of misinformation which surrounds these germs. The majority of viruses are incapable of reproducing on their own; they must infect other cells. They thrive by attacking and invading a host's cells, reproducing within them. Thus, they parasitize the cells and organs.

Viruses are invaders, a kind of intracellular parasite. They greatly damage the body's cellular infrastructure. Disease results from cell damage and death. The cells sacrifice their genetic machinery and nutrients to support the viruses' voracious metabolic needs.

The danger with viruses is, in fact, related to their size. These invaders are able to evade the immune defenses, stealthily infecting the cells. They are created to attack. For survival they thrive on human or animal cells. Without human or animal cells— living cells in real living bodies—there would be no viral infections.

Viruses possess a highly sophisticated mechanism for invading human cells. Once they gain entrance, they are difficult to destroy. Within these cells they set into motion their genetic machinery, which, in fact, overtakes the cell's own apparatus. The virus 'tells' the cell's genes precisely what to do, that is to make new viruses.

Only a massive immune response is able to cleanse the cells of these invaders. This is a primary purpose of fever, since such high body temperatures help kill intracellular viruses. Fever should never be purposely repressed. It represents an active immune response. It should be assisted, that is through natural substances which kill viruses. Once such viruses are killed, the fever dissipates.

Spice oils are highly viricidal, which means they aggressively kill these germs. Extracts of wild spices, that is the essential spice oils, are potent virus killers, so potent that they can eliminate fever in minutes. It is the mechanism of action which is critical. Repressing the fever, that is *repressing the symptom of fever*, is harmful. Causing the fever to dissipate *by treating the cause, that is by killing the virus*, is entirely different. This is what wild spice extracts, such as Oregacyn and Oreganol, achieve. They halt the agonizing symptoms of colds, flu, sinus attacks, bronchitis, and pneumonia without any harm, in fact, with immeasurable benefit. Regarding the aforementioned diseases the use of a combined therapy: the Oregacyn multiple-spice capsules, along with the Oreganol oil, which is, ideally, taken under the tongue, leads to a dramatic improvement. The duration of epidemic flu and colds, as well as chronic respiratory conditions, can be reduced by up to 90%. What might prove to be a week-long illness is reduced to a day or two, while a potential three week sickness is cut to a few days. Chronic diseases, which have lasted for months and/or years, are eliminated in mere days. What's more, the individual during the course of the disease remains relatively vital and even functional—even in many cases capable of carrying a full or nearly full workload. That is evidence of the potent medicinal powers of wild mountainous spices: the medicines of Almighty God.

Chapter 3
The Diseases

The number of infectious diseases which are striking humanity is frightening. There are a greater number of epidemics afflicting the human race now than ever before in history. In the past civilizations had to contend with a single epidemic, not dozens, as is occurring today. The fact is there are a greater number of uncontrollable infectious diseases attacking the human race than can be listed in this book. This is a frightening fact. However, the most significant of these epidemics are listed. Continuously, it seems, a new infection emerges, threatening to disable and destroy human populations. Diseases seemingly emerge spontaneously, which are destructive to the human race. This is far from a casual issue: it is an absolute fact. What's more, these are not merely acts of nature. People are dying, largely as a result of human meddling. AIDS, Mad Cow, West Nile, Lyme, mutant bacteria, encephalitis, and systemic fungus are directly tied to human corruptions. Thus, the human race is enduring a sort of self-destruction, largely due to bizarre infectious diseases.

Today, every hospital is a danger zone. What's more, many doctors' offices are, from a microbial point of view, equally toxic. In these facilities drug-resistant mutants are prolific, potent genetically altered germs capable of rapidly infecting humans. This is where sick people congregate, and, thus, it is where the pathogens reside.

Drug-resistant mutants are pathogens of the most diabolical degree. These mutated germs have altered structural properties which make them virtually indestructible—the human immune system can no longer resist them. Many of these altered germs attack by stealth: they invade and destroy the tissues before the immune system can react. The fact is many of these organisms are so stealth-like that they utterly evade the immune system. They are even capable of striking directly into its power-base: the lymph tissue and the white blood cells themselves. This is a frightening capacity. If unchecked, such germs will destroy much of the human race, that is unless the proper defenses are raised or, rather, unless precise cures are achieved.

The Western world is the progenitor of frightening man-made infections. There are a greater number of germ zones in the United States than many Third World countries. This is in part due to bizarre sexual practices, including the rampant practices of homosexuality. Sexual promiscuity, including prostitution, is another factor. The fact is there is an attitude in the United States that a person has a "right" to engage in any sexual activity he or she desires. The statistics are ominous: some 40% of all men engage at some point in their lives in secretive extramarital sex, and nearly 60% of all teens become sexually active before marriage. Obviously, this leads to the spread of a wide range of diseases. This is so-called casual sex, that is the direct, invasive contact of body parts with individuals unknown.

The term adultery is descriptive. People have regarded primarily its spiritual implications. It is derived from adulterate, which means to corrupt—to contaminate. It means to render unfit for use. This is precisely what is achieved. Through adulterous sex the human body is contaminated, physically, socially, and spiritually. What's more, there is always an unknowing, that is innocent, victim. For instance, a man has so-called casual sex with a 'stranger.' Then, he has sex with his partner. Thus, the partner is adulterated, that is contaminated. What's more, the adulterated individual is a victim, who could develop a life-threatening disease, having no clue regarding its source. The victimization fails to end there. Evidence exists that any sexually transmitted disease is also transmitted to offspring: through the womb. Then, such contaminated children continue to spread the infestation to their future heirs. The victimization afflicts the gene pool forever. Thus, the adulteration is thorough and complete. The degree of pain inflicted from a single act of indiscretion—a single act of lust—is beyond measure. This is why in scripture it is condemned to the highest degree.

In the Western world as a consequence of sexual excesses there exist a wide variety of epidemics. Chlamydia, genital herpes, genital warts, hepatitis, genital yeast infections, trichomonas, and gonorrhea—even certain forms of syphilis— are rampant epidemics. All could be prevented by curbing sexual promiscuity.

There is even a more dire practice: bizarre, that is unnatural, sexual acts. Such unnatural practices greatly spread disease and create horrifying infection zones: gay clubs, bars, and bath-houses, where fulminant, in fact, life-threatening infections breed. From these the infections can spread into the general public. In essence the gay institutions act as microbial breweries and from here epidemics can be seeded.

Few people discuss this connection. They fear the aggressive gay lobby, which, apparently, systematically attacks any "detractors". Yet, this is far from a political or even social attack on gays. Rather, it is a physiological fact. There would occur a major reduction in sexually transmitted diseases, that is if normal physiology were adhered to: male-female sex. These physiological partners are correctly suited for the sex act. This is not the case, for instance, with male-to-male sex. The fact is the latter is not even sex at all. It is an aberration. Men have no natural receptacle to receive the penis. In contrast, in women the vagina precisely receives it.

There is another even more diabolical aberration: human-to-animal sex. Here, men and women contaminate themselves with potentially aggressive animal germs by direct inoculation.

Consider the AIDS virus and the devastation it has caused. This was originally spread via homosexual practices. The point is, physiologically, men are designed to have sex with women: in the vaginal tract. Sex acts, where men force the penis into the rectums of other men, or, for that matter, women, is a violation of nature. The fact that this violates normal anatomy and physiology is undeniable. The result is disease, which may be, ultimately, transmitted to the innocent.

Ideally, gay men must consider a simple fact: it is physiologically normal to have sex with women. What's more, physiologically, such individuals are men, not women. Thus, why engage in sex acts with what is the physiological and anatomical opposite? This is also the correct spiritual and social relationship, that is man with woman. It is also the normal relationship, that is the natural love instinct—the way the eye and heart are naturally drawn: for a man towards a woman and visa versa. The fact is it would be to the individual's benefit, including the so-called gay man, to pursue such a normal relationship.The benefits are legion and include better health, greater satisfaction, a happier being and a longer life. For people who deem themselves gay consider a simple fact: the dire misery and agony of dying of AIDS or a similar catastrophic disease, all due to violations against nature. Due to their high rate of infectious diseases gays have a lower life expectancy than the norm. Thus, by adopting a physiological relationship between man and woman, as demanded by nature, great benefits are gained and catastrophes, as well as premature death, would be avoided.

Rectal sex spreads germs. The feces contain untold trillions of pathogens. When performing rectal sex, there is no means to be safeguarded. Human feces is highly caustic and is a vile substance. Thus, there is no safe means to perform such an act. Within the rectum the penis acts as a device for spreading the germs. Its forceful movement propels fecal contents against gravity, leading to retrograde fecal motion. In other words, the feces is pushed upwards toward the stomach. This leads to septic infections in the upper digestive tract. Certainly, ulcerative colitis and Crohn's disease may be a consequence of repeated acts of rectal sex. What's more, while condoms may offer a degree of protection, inevitably, when there is exposure to feces, there will be contamination. Certain sub-microscopic particles, such as viruses and mycoplasmas, may penetrate the barrier. Fecal material may regurgitate over it. Thus, there is no way to have "safe" or sterile rectal sex. Since feces is caustic, that is highly penetrating, it can penetrate through even a barrier. Bile is an emulsifier, and the feces is rife with it. Condoms are readily penetrated by it. What's more, through openings or wounds in the skin contamination may inadvertently occur. What's more, regarding direct contact of the penis in the rectum, regardless of any washing, there is contamination. This is because the feces is forcefully propelled into the urethra, rapidly leading to sepsis. The kidneys are infected, and fecal contents enter the bloodstream. In homosexuals this is the more likely cause of AIDS or AIDS-like syndromes than a government conspiracy.

Sepsis breeds further sepsis. Unnatural sex acts, especially between men, not only harm the perpetrators but cause harm throughout civilization. The body can only handle a minor degree of septic assault. Gay practices cause septic overload. The vastness of the germ exposure—billions or even trillions of germs per session—overtaxes the immune system's abilities. Ultimately, due to such an inordinate degree of infection it degenerates, and fulminant disease results.

Direct contact with human feces will cause disease, especially if the contact is repetitive. The feces contain untold millions of species of germs, many of which are highly pathogenic. It is meant to be held in the colon, so it can be expelled as waste. If such material is reintroduced into the body—that is if it gains entrance into the upper digestive tract, urethra, and/or bloodstream—there can only be one consequence: serious disease, perhaps death. People act as if it is their right to engage in such acts. Yet, by doing so such individuals place the entire human civilization at risk.

The human being has been imbued with a natural attraction to the opposite sex, which is undeniable. There is no such natural attraction between men, that is for physical, in other words, sexual, love. For instance, the hormone systems of males and females vary dramatically. These hormone systems are strictly for created the opposite sex attraction. In the animal kingdom females enter estrus, which attracts males. The smell of male hormones repels other males, in fact, creates the opposite of love: aggression. For humans women exude hormone secretions, which cause a corresponding secretion in males. There is no such hormone secretion causing males to attract males or females to attract females. There is no natural attraction to cause a man to make love to a man or a woman to do so to another woman. Thus, the homosexual propensity, as well as the act itself, violates nature. If such individuals, who are in violation of nature, would consider a simplistic approach: converting to the natural way and pursuing relationships with women—as love and soul mates—such individuals would greatly benefit, emotionally, spiritually, and physically. The human race would benefit by a significant reduction in the spread of disease. Uncountable lives of the innocent, as well as the perpetrators themselves, would be saved. The fact is abnormal sex leads to disease not only in the perpetrators but also in the general population.

Rampant homosexuality spreads disease, causing the deaths of the innocent. The fact is it is far from so-called gay rights for the individual to do as he/she pleases. By doing so such individuals place other individuals at risk, in fact, entire civilizations. Thus, bizarre sexual behaviors must be curbed, that is for the sake of the perpetrator as well as all humankind. Gays have no "right" to be gay. By violating nature they destroy not only themselves but also the lives of the innocent: the unsuspecting individual, who engages in sex with the contaminated or the blood recipient, whose health is wrongfully and violently devastated or who perhaps dies as a result of homosexual-related infections. Thus, wanton so-called free sex is far from free: it costs enormously, that is in human lives and agony. The fact is when homosexual men give blood, they essentially seed disease within the population. The hepatitis C epidemic can largely be traced to transfusions, which, again, is directly tied to homosexual contamination. Thus, there is an enormous cost of free sex: the cost of premature death and uncountable human agony.

There is another major debacle which afflicts the Western world: drug-resistant germs. These germs are the result of the overuse of antibiotics. Originally killers of hospitalized patients, now these germs are commonly found in outpatient clinics and doctor's offices, where they infect the unsuspecting. Millions of Americans yearly become contaminated with these mutants, leading to severe infections, diseases, tissue damage, and even death. According to *JAMA* a minimum of 250,000 people lose their lives in hospitals every year from antibiotic-induced disease: sepsis by drug-resistant germs. Yet, there are uncountable others who are direly sickened, losing their health and even their limbs due to these freakish germs. People die excruciatingly painful deaths from infections, which could be cured. Yet, there are no medical cures for drug-resistant germs. Only nature offers such cures. It may require massive amounts of natural substances to eradicate them. Yet, only nature offers the power to destroy such toxic germs, where the synthetic world remains impotent. It provides the only options, since drugs have utterly failed. Thus, natural substances, made by a power which is unfathomable, that is which is beyond the human realm, offer hope for humankind against plagues of its own making. In other words, almighty God can help us; humans are unable to. A study by Georgetown University provides the proof. Here, animals infected with drug-resistant staph were treated with a potent drug, Vancomycin, as well as a potent type of wild oregano, that is P73 Oreganol. Half the drug-treated mice survived, but so did half the Oreganol P73-treated ones. This is an impressive result, since for drug-resistant staph infections Vancomycin is the drug of last resort. Thus, the natural compound was equivalent to the drug. What's more, the natural compound proved superior to the synthetic. The researchers made an interesting discovery. The survivors on the oregano oil were healthier than those given the drugs. This is what is meant by the potential for cure: natural substances offer the ability to assist the healing process, whereas drugs often cause irreversible toxicity. What's more, natural compounds can be given in relatively large doses, again, without toxicity, whereas the synthetics must be administered with great care due to the risk for organ damage as well as death. Yearly, drugs kill tens of thousands of people. Herbal medicines and whole foods heal them, in fact, reverse the damage.

These are preventable deaths. This is because there are natural ways to kill such germs. Plus, the immune system can be boosted, so it can eradicate such infections. Even in hospitalized patients if the proper approach were taken by giving immune-boosting foods and supplements, dramatic cures could be achieved. Thus, people are dying due to ignorance and neglect. What's more, there are a number of natural medicines which kill mutant germs. Oregacyn P73 is the most powerful, as well as proven, of these. Plus, natural antibiotics, such as the Oregacyn, fail to induce such fatal, that is drug-resistant, infections. Rather, they eradicate them.

AIDS

Few people seem to be interested in this epidemic; it has almost become as if passé. This is because it is not as devastating to the general population as was once thought. Yet, for those who do contract it nothing could be more devastating. It remains a disease contracted largely through direct sexual contact, blood transfusions, and IV drug use.

A kind of low-grade AIDS may strike. This is an immunodeficiency due to vaccinations, which are contaminated with AIDS-like viruses. Thus, there are, in fact, tens of millions of individuals who suffer from a kind of immunosuppression, a pseudo-AIDS.

Then, there is fulminant AIDS as well as HIV. These diseases occur primarily in high risk groups, mainly homosexuals, drug addicts, prostitutes, and newborn children of the sexually active. However, untold millions also contract it through having sex with the infected. What's more, in Africa the disease is epidemic. Here, sexual contact alone fails to account for the spread. There is a direct tie to vaccination as a cause. Regarding women, blacks and Hispanics are the preponderance of victims:

some 70%. The same is true of infants and children: 78% are black and Hispanics.

Yet, this is far from a disease of the poor. This is because for the majority AIDS is contracted via sex. While there are innocent victims, such as hemophiliacs and vaccine recipients, the majority of cases occur in the sexually active, that is those who have transient sexual relationships. Thus, in many respects AIDS is a preventable disease. By adhering to the divine code—the law of never going near a casual sexual relationship, regardless of the temptation—catastrophes can be avoided. Especially in the teenage years with raging hormones this may be easier said than done. However, the consequences may be dire: a slow agonizing death by a virtually incurable disease. What's more, teenagers in particular must understand a certain fact: having sex with a stranger is no act of "conquering." It is never "cool." It is an absolute danger zone. What's more, there is no need to "practice" sex. It is a natural and rather forgiving act, that is when it occurs under the proper and "legitimate" pretext, all usually transpires without incident. In other words, there is no need to feel "embarrassed" due to a lack of experience. When it happens, it virtually always proceeds without embarrassment.

Homosexuals develop a fulminant kind of AIDS. This is the classic case of septic contamination, where a wide range of germs infect the tissues. The sexual practices of such individuals are responsible for this contamination. The degree of infection is vast: Candida, herpes, klebsiella, staph, strep, amoebas, worms, pneumocystis, blastocystis, cytomegalovirus, hepatitis viruses, HIV, and uncountable others. A mere look at such individuals, who are often ill appearing—pale, clammy, and septic-appearing—tells all. The sepsis violates all regions of the body, leading to total immune collapse. The results are dire: premature death from rampant infections, the AIDS virus itself, and/or cancer.

Fulminant respiratory infections, such as SARS, are spread by close contact. The fact is SARS is a highly contagious disease, perhaps one of the most contagious ever known. Sexual contact is a means of spread. San Francisco, with its large gay population, is a logical source for the spread. Here, gays participate in promiscuous sexual encounters, quickly disseminating infections. It is well known that diseases spread rapidly among homosexuals. For instance, in Los Angeles mutant Staph aureus, resistant to all antibiotics, broke out and spread rapidly among a group of homosexuals. From here it is feared that it will spread uncontrollably within the general public. This is precisely what is now occurring. In southern California this staph is attacking people unmercifully. Suddenly, people are developing bizarre infections in their fingers, hands, arms, and legs. It is mutant staph. This mutated germ is resistant to all antibiotics. In fact, the giving of antibiotics accelerates both its invasive powers and its spread. Yet, it is a simple fact: multiple sexual encounters, particularly anal sex, encourages the spread of germs, including mutant staph as well as E. coli. If a person inserts his penis in the rectum, it becomes contaminated with feces. This is mere common sense that such an act must lead to the spread of germs. Such feces contains billions of germs, many of which are highly pathogenic, that is dangerous. Then, if the individual has further sex, especially with unsuspecting individuals, the fecal germs, as well as any germs which grow in the perpetrator's sperm, are further spread. This leads to fulminant epidemics. Thus, it is impossible to perform hygienic or "safe" sex within the feces-contaminated rectum.

Perhaps even more diabolical certain individuals have sex with animals. This results in the spread of animal viruses, bacteria, and parasites, which readily devastate the body. There is evidence to indicate that AIDS was spread, perhaps originated, in this manner. What's more, the AIDS virus has been directly correlated with another infection: fecal amoebas. Once these amoebas fully invade, they greatly depress the immune system, leaving the body vulnerable to AIDS viruses. Gay individuals, who aggressively perform rectal sex, may harbor untold billions of these parasites in their blood. This creates such a vast immune suppression that virtually any infection can gain momentum.

The issue is germs, such as mutant staph, HIV, and the SARS virus, are highly contagious. Close contact is the primary means of spread. Intimate sexual contact spreads infection, leading to potentially fatal infestations. This is far from an attack against any single group. Rather, it is merely the facts. Because of constant close contact, often with total strangers, homosexuals are a major source of the spread of pandemic diseases. It must be reiterated that certain individuals, including a significant number of homosexuals, have sex with animals. What's more, they may engage in such sex acts while intoxicated by drugs. Thus, they may be unaware of the exact nature of the sex act. Then, in some cases while fully contaminated they have sex with their partners or spouses. This greatly accelerates the dissemination of pandemic germs. Super-breeders are created. Animal pathogens, including highly aggressive viruses capable of disabling the immune system, invade the victims. It is well known that dogs carry retroviruses, the same family as the AIDS virus. Could AIDS originate from dog viruses? Certainly, such viruses are highly immunosuppressive and are capable of neutralizing, in fact, obliterating, the immune cells.

There is no question that people who have sex with animals retain the animal pathogens. Such germs become residents of the body, infecting, for instance, the kidneys, blood, and sexual organs. When sex acts are performed, the infection is spread. In particular, homosexuals may engage in sexual encounters with multiple individuals, even in the same day. Thus, the homosexual population represents the most ripe breeding ground for aggressive, highly destructive germs. Prostitutes, as well as highly active heterosexuals, may also serve as the breeding ground for such germs. The fact is anyone who engages in sex with multiple individuals will readily become infected with life-threatening germs.

It is all for such a short encounter: such a temporary pleasure. Yet, it puts the individual's life at risk as well as all his/her future sexual contacts.

Regarding SARS, as well as AIDS, in the United States the San Francisco Bay area was one of the epicenters for the infection. It is likely that the epidemic will spread, largely from San Francisco to ultimately strike every region in the country. Much of the spread could be prevented, that is if homosexuals would adopt the normal, physiological practice: having women as their sexual partners rather than men and/or animals. This natural practice, which follows the normal anatomy of the male and female, would dramatically minimize the spread of disease. This would help eliminate the highly dangerous practice of anal sex. The latter greatly spreads infectious diseases. The fact is anal sex is highly traumatic, regardless of the encounter.

The rectum is different structurally than the vagina. This is because the vagina is constructed to accommodate the penis; the rectum fails to do so. When such a hardened object enters the rectum, the latter is traumatized. The rectal walls are readily torn. The penis fails to properly fit there. In contrast, the vagina readily accommodates it. The rectum has no ability to expand. This leads to the seepage of fecal matter, as well as semen, into the bloodstream, which causes a wide range of disorders. There is no question that fecal contamination played a major role in the spread of AIDS. In this country such a disease has caused untold death and devastation. Blood products were contaminated with AIDS-causing germs, further spreading the infection, perhaps globally. The diabolical sexual tendencies of homosexuals not only lead to their own harm but also have impacted people globally, causing an unprecedented degree of human harm.

Consider the spread of AIDS, which began in homosexual flight attendants visiting Haiti. These were the first cases: male flight attendants from Air France, who developed AIDS as a result of homosexual sex acts. Other original cases occurred in San Francisco Bay, where an outbreak of amoebic infection among homosexuals coincided with the AIDS outbreak. amoebic infections strictly arise from fecal contact. As a result of the aberrant sexual practices of the few, millions of innocent individuals have become infected. Blood has become tainted, causing the infection of untold other innocents. The blood today is far from safe: gays are infected with far more than merely the AIDS virus. Any blood that has as its source an active homosexual is bound to transmit disease, particularly other unknown animal viruses exist as contaminants.

People clamor for so-called gay rights. Others claim a state of indifference. Yet, what about the rights of the innocent, who contract this plague due to the vile deeds of the few? What about the infant who contracts AIDS from an infected mother: a mother who was infected by her bisexual husband? Or, the blood transfusion recipient, who develops this disease due to homosexual-donated blood? Homosexual sex acts are responsible for the deaths of hundreds of thousands, perhaps millions, of innocent victims yearly. The suffering, death, and despair is beyond count. Aren't these the rights that should be the focus—the rights of the innocent victims, the rights of even innocent babies, whose futures have been destroyed—rather than the supposed rights of the perpetrator?

Contaminated sex clinics must be shut down. Certainly, by the government bizarre sex acts should never be encouraged. Government approval of homosexual sex, that is by allowing marriage licenses, must be challenged, that is based upon the impugning of the rights of the innocent. Government support of deviant behaviors must be halted. Otherwise, this nation will be subjected to doom: the same doom that afflicted prior corrupt civilizations. Regarding moral or social issues the government has no right to mandate laws. Only almighty God can do so. Even if the government fails to abide by the divine code for social and health reasons it must take action. For sanitary reasons it must create regulations, that is the regulations necessary to protect its citizens, who are being harmed, killed, and victimized due to the passions of the few. The fact is by supporting homosexuality the government becomes an accessory to a crime: the infection and ultimate death of innocent individuals.

AIDS began in homosexuals. This is indisputable. It spread from such individuals to other people, including heterosexuals, that is people who only have sex with the opposite sex. These are the internationally recognized facts. So, how could there be any other cause, that is other than homosexual practices?

This is far from a condemnation of individual people. Rather, it is a condemnation against a specific practice, which violates all norms—which directly violates the natural laws and which, therefore, places human beings at risk, rather, the entire human race. It is also a warning to such people, that is to change their destructive habits before they destroy themselves.

Incredibly, people often become homosexual because they are angry. The fact is they are angry because they were created as men instead of women (or visa versa). Or, they use being homosexual as a means of "control", which is often violent.

Regarding the consequences of aberrant sex acts people should be educated. They should realize the risks, that is for self destruction. They should realize that if they continue to commit such practices, they will sicken themselves. Homosexual encounters, using the rectum as the conduit, are highly traumatic. The spread of infection is unavoidable. The fact is homosexuals must realize that they are harming themselves, perhaps irreparably, by such a practice. Plus, education should be achieved against having sex with animals. Such practices not only traumatize the animals but also those who perpetrate such acts. It reduces the individual morally to the lowest level. The animal viruses readily attack the immune system, ultimately destroying it. What's more, the brain is attacked by such viruses, which further destabilize mental function. Furthermore, the animals become victims and, therefore, spread disease—human infections—among their own kind. Even the psyche of the animals is disturbed: they are tormented for life, since they have been forced to practice bizarre acts, which violate their instincts.

Animal viruses and other pathogens aggressively infect humans. The result is the destruction of health. AIDS may well be an animal virus—as well as other animal pathogens—which has mutated to infect humans. Its source could readily be various dog viruses. Having sex with dogs is a relatively common practice, performed both by homosexuals and heterosexuals. Particularly when intoxicated homosexuals perform a wide range of unnatural acts, including having sex with animals, particularly dogs. Dog semen is fully contaminated with viruses, including types which attack the brain, spinal cord, and immune cells. This is a far more likely source of the AIDS epidemic than, for instance, as has been recently popularized, a deliberate government conspiracy.

Treatment protocol

AIDS is due to septic contamination of the blood and internal organs. Thus, an antiseptic approach is necessary. Take the highly antiseptic Oreganol oil of oregano, five or more drops under the tongue several times daily. Take also the Oregacyn, two capsules three times daily Also, take the Oreganol P73 Juice, one ounce two or three times daily. Wild rosemary and sage inhibit the AIDS virus. Take the sage/rosemary formula, Neuroloft capsules, three capsules twice daily. Also, on any suspicious lesion apply the Oreganol cream as often as needed. SuperStrength Oreganol is a potent remedy for this condition. In tough cases large amounts must be taken such as a dropperful under the tongue several times daily. This therapy may be taken as often as every few minutes. Also, when taking megadoses of oregano take also healthy bacteria, that is the Health-Bac, two heaping teaspoons in a warm glass of water at night before bedtime. This will also help normalize any toxicity of the gut. What's more, to detoxify the internal organs take the GreensFlush, 40 or more drops twice daily. Follow this protocol for at least 90 days. For hepatitis C also add the LivaClenz, two or three capsules daily with full meals. The activity of the latter is increased by extra virgin olive oil. When taking LivaClenz, take it with a tablespoon or two of extra virgin olive oil. Infla-eez, a potent source of protein-digesting enzymes, may also prove valuable: take three twice daily.

Food poisoning

The food supply has largely been contaminated. Incredibly, some 100 million Americans contract food poisoning yearly. Many of these develop intractable diseases: several hundred die. Regarding this epidemic the overuse of antibiotics is largely to blame. However, imported foods, especially fruits and vegetables, are also a major culprit. Growing practices may include the use of contaminated fertilizer, which may not be properly washed off. Animal wastes are applied directly to the soil and growing plants and are rarely composted. Lack of proper food hygiene by laborers, as well as consumers, is also a considerable risk. Here, the food may have originally been hygienic but is later contaminated by the handler, who fails to attend to proper hygiene, especially hand-washing. The consumer may err by failing to thoroughly wash the food. This is common; people somehow believe that if it comes from the commercial market it is safe; no further cleaning or decontaminating is necessary. Incredibly, people frequently fail to wash their fresh vegetables and fruit, even salad. The result is untold millions of cases of food poisoning. The fact is there are potentially millions of germs lodged within, for instance, a head of dirty lettuce or spinach. If such vegetables are served unwashed, which is common in certain restaurants, food poisoning is likely.

Food poisoning is more common than the flu. It is seemingly less ominous than most diseases, since the majority of people recover from it. Yet, do they fully recover? Lingering side effects are common, some of which are serious. For instance, camphylobacter may cause inflammatory colitis, gallbladder disorders, muscular wasting, and the bizarre paralysis condition known as Guillian-Barré syndrome. Shigella can cause severe reactive colitis as well as arthritis and liver disorders. E. coli can result in severe bladder, kidney, liver, and intestinal disorders. It can even cause a potentially fatal toxic shock syndrome. A debilitating type of arthritis, as well as liver/gallbladder disease, results from salmonella infection. Thus, after a severe bout of food poisoning many people are left weakened for life. Here again such individuals are victims of septic exposure. Only proper hygiene and food handling practices can curb the incidence of this epidemic. Natural antiseptics are also crucial. They can largely prevent food poisoning. For travelers a natural antiseptic "kit" is invaluable. This kit consists of a bottle of Oreganol P73, along with Oregacyn, the latter being an antibiotic-like multiple spice extract, plus the natural bacterial supplement, Health-Bac. The oil is ideal for use under the tongue, for instance, for treating and/or preventing head and neck disorders, including sinus, allergy, and cold/flu attacks, plus it is invaluable for use topically. Here, it is useful for a wide range of disorders and injuries, including cuts, abrasions, halting of hemorrhage, burns, sunburn, venomous bites, insect bites, warts, and rashes. This is a lifesaving kit. The regular use of this kit will essentially prevent the dire events typical of international travel and cuisine. Eat to your heart's desire (but do not gorge), however, take the components of the kit on a regular basis.

Virtually any germ can cause food poisoning, including a wide range of bacteria, viruses, and parasites. In the United States bacteria appear to be the most likely culprits. Salmonella toxicity is perhaps the most common type of food poisoning, followed by E. coli, staph, listeria, and shigella. Increasingly, parasites are implicated in bouts of food poisoning. In the Third World parasites are the primary aggressors. Viruses usually cause a less severe form of food poisoning. For example, the Norwalk virus, which is, in fact, a kind of intestinal flu, causes relatively self-limiting syndrome, manifested by fever, cramping, vomiting, and diarrhea. It usually lasts only about 48 hours. In contrast parasites can cause illnesses that can last weeks, perhaps a lifetime. Certain viruses can also cause severe food poisoning, for instance, the hepatitis viruses. Regarding the latter their direct actions upon liver health are well known. The virus aggressively attacks this organ, destroying uncountable liver cells and resulting in the condition known as yellow jaundice. This happens yearly in the United States, where people contract potentially fatal hepatitis from restaurant food.

Treatment protocol

Raw unprocessed honey is highly effective in reversing food poisoning. This is especially true for bacterial and/or viral diarrhea. Oil of wild oregano is also highly effective. A combination of crude raw honey, such as the wild oregano and/or thistle honeys, with a few drops of Oreganol is highly effective for halting this condition. Note: usually, such honeys are only available via mail-order. These are rare honeys, made by bees in mountainous areas and are unique, since the bees are never fed sugar. They are exceptionally pure, because they are harvested directly from the mountains. Thus, such honeys are safe for use in all age groups. The mountain-raised honeys, which are derived from wild plants, are the ideal medicinal types: they are medicines as well as foods. To order call 1-800-243-5242 or in Canada 1-866-776-6550. For every tablespoon of crude raw honey add five to ten drops of oil of wild oregano (i.e. Oreganol). Regarding the latter do not use cheap imitations, which are usually derived from Spanish thyme, which is inedible. A number of manufacturers are currently bottling Spanish thyme under the generic name "oil of wild oregano," or "oil of oregano," or "Origanum vulgare." Such products fail to even contain oregano oil, instead containing the highly inferior Origanum vulgare, farm-raised marjarom, and/or Spanish thyme. Do not use such counterfeit oils. Instead, buy the 100% wild material, that is the Oreganol, which is derived from the edible spice. This oil is extensively researched, both for safety and efficacy.

Labels which read "Origanum vulgare" are usually a sign of inferior quality. This is because under this category there are over 80 different plants. The category includes not only farm-raised types but also the inedible Thymus capitus. Avoid any product which makes such label claims. Rather, the label should state that the product is researched and that only 100% wild oregano is used. The fact is counterfeit oregano oils are unfit for human consumption, since they are derived from the often adulterated Thymus capitus. The latter may even be rectified, that is refined, which, in fact, concentrates its toxicity. Strictly avoid the consumption of such products. For instance, in Canada a survey was done on oil of oregano products. There were at least a dozen such products on the shelf, incredibly, many of which were recommended for internal use. Yet, none are safe for internal consumption, because none were derived from the edible spice. Only use oregano oil guaranteed to be from the edible wild spice. The key is wild spice, never farm-raised. Brands which qualify for such a distinction include, in the United States, Vitamin Shoppe and North American Herb & Spice (i. e. Oreganol) and in Canada, Oreganol, as well as Vivitas.

In food poisoning the gut is already damaged. The body needs herbs that will aid in the cure, not irritants. The Oreganol is a highly sophisticated product. It is safe for use during food poisoning, as are the OregaMax capsules. Regarding the latter it is a digestive tonic similar to the old-fashioned digestive bitters. It is also a general immune booster. Also, in terms of antiseptic action do not depend upon cheap honeys. Usually, such honeys offer only minimal potency. This is because to make such inexpensive honeys beekeepers feed the bees sugar, which greatly weakens their immune systems. A honey derived from sugar-fed bees is never fit as a medicine. Such feeding significantly lessens the quality, minimizing medicinal properties. Do not expect medicinal results from such honeys. Also, as an antidiarrheal and digestive tonic take Health-Bac, one teaspoon daily. Health-bac is a highly effective natural bacterial supplement, ideal for driving out noxious pathogens, while re-establishing the function of the gut. I have used this very successfully when traveling overseas. Drink only water and fresh juice. Consume only the clear broths of soups. Thus, a resting of the gut is the ideal means of achieving a more rapid cure. In summary a simple protocol for eradicating food poisoning is: wild oregano or thistle honey with added oregano oil and Health-Bac. For resistant cases try also the natural antibiotic capsule, that is the Oregacyn, one or two capsules every few hours.

Anthrax

The likelihood for an anthrax attack is remote, and natural transmission is restricted to areas where livestock is raised. Yet, there remains a possibility of infection, plus there is no medical treatment. Untreated, the fatality rate for anthrax is nearly 100%.

Anthrax is rare. The likelihood of Americans contracting this disease, especially city-dwellers, is remote. However, as a result of the release in 2001 in the United States of weaponized anthrax, which was, apparently, sent to certain dissidents, a number of people died. Short of the release of weaponized material there is a greater risk of getting struck by lightning than contracting anthrax. Even so, an outbreak of naturally occurring or weaponized anthrax could occur in North America. Plus, since there is no medical cure alternatives must be discussed. So-called terrorist attacks with anthrax would be an effective means for eliminating political enemies.

There are three forms of this disease: the skin form, the lung form, and the intestinal form. The skin form develops primarily in the exposed areas of the skin, usually at the area of a cut, scratch, or abrasion. After a short incubation, about two days, the lesion begins as a small red elevation, which looks similar to a mosquito bite. It usually itches. As the lesion evolves it becomes swollen. In the center a vesicle consisting of clear fluid develops, and nearby other vesicles may develop. Then, in that center the tissue begins to die, with the typical development of a black lesion. Lymph nodes in the region may swell, which can be painful but, interestingly, the lesion is non-painful. As the infection passes from the lymph nodes to the blood, fever and chills may develop. The mortality rate for this type of anthrax is 20%.

The lung type is due to the inhalation of anthrax spores. Other than the release of weaponized anthrax there are few if any cases yearly of this form of anthrax in the United States. The mechanism is that once the spores are inhaled, they are absorbed by the white blood cells. These cells carry the spores to the lungs' lymph glands, where surviving bacteria multiply in vast quantities. This multiplication causes the lungs to become obstructed, leading to respiratory failure and death. The mortality of this type of anthrax is over 90%. Symptoms of inhalation anthrax include a flu-like presentation, muscle aches, dry cough, and a frequent sensation of chest pressure as well as a sense of suffocating. Fever and chills usually develop, along with sweating and shortness of breath. Ultimately, cyanosis develops. Intestinal anthrax is caused through eating contaminated food. Today, this type of anthrax is exceptionally rare.

Treatment protocol

There is little that can be done for severe respiratory anthrax, that is the type caused by the weaponized spore. The federal government disallows making claims for cure. Even so, spice extracts offer potent germicidal powers. Research in Egypt shows that certain spice oils, such as oils of cumin and cinnamon, which are found in Oregacyn, kill anthrax-like germs. A preliminary study by Georgetown University is encouraging: oil of wild oregano (P73) partially destroyed anthrax bacilli in the test tube. The Pentagon itself is aware of this and has recommended oil of oregano for certain troops. Tests by Celsus Labs prove that oil of wild oregano, as well as oil of wild cumin, both of which are key ingredients of Oregacyn, directly inhibits the growth of this germ.

The medical treatment for anthrax is the drug, Cipro. However, the Oreganol and Oregacyn offer adjunctive treatment, which could mean the difference between life and death. Aggressive doses are the key: in the event of serious infection take the Oregacyn, as many as three capsules every hour or half hour, with food or heavy juice such as tomato, V-8, or carrot juice. Also, take the oil under the tongue, five or more drops on the hour or half hour.

Candidiasis

This is one of the greatest plagues afflicting Westerners. Candida is a yeast, which normally lives in the human intestine as well as mouth and skin. It is known as a commensal organism, meaning it lives in a balance normally in the body, along with similar native germs. When out of balance, it causes significant disruption of body chemistry, ultimately leading to disease.

Candida only overgrows as a result of human meddling. Poor diet creates imbalances, which can lead to the infection. In particular, a diet excessively rich in refined sugars and starches stimulates its growth. The average American consumes some 150 pounds of sugar yearly, which will automatically result in yeast overgrowth. The consumption of heavily processed and sugar-infested foods, such as doughnuts, sweet rolls, cakes, muffins, pies, commercial breads, sugary breakfast cereals, granola bars, buns, rolls, pop, fruit drinks, cookies, and candies, greatly increases the sugar content within the blood. As a result Candida flourishes. Only a relatively small amount of sugar, a mere teaspoon, is sufficient to accelerate candida growth.

To eliminate this infection it is critical to change the diet. Foods containing refined sugars must be avoided. The carbohydrate intake must be curtailed. The diet must consist of naturally or organically raised meat products, organic milk/egg products, wild fish, fruit, vegetables, and healthy complex carbohydrates. Regarding the latter baked potatoes, wild rice, brown rice, lentils, beans, and coarse whole grains are acceptable. Invasive medical therapy, as well as drugs, is equally important as is diet in causing this disease. The fact is candidiasis is largely a medically induced disease. Antibiotic therapy is a major cause. A mere course of a potent antibiotic can induce it, as can a course of cortisone, that is Prednisone. Consider the people who have had numerous courses of antibiotics. Certainly, they suffer from the systemic infection. What's more, radiation therapy, as well as consistent medical x-rays, is a major factor which creates the infection.

Candidiasis is the great mimicker. Physicians may find it difficult to diagnose the infection. The fact is, frequently, it is misdiagnosed as various conditions such as fibromyalgia, chronic fatigue syndrome, arthritis, lupus, hypothyroidism, irritable bowel syndrome, Crohn's disease, ulcerative colitis, Sjogren's syndrome, ankylosing spondylitis, esophagitis, endometriosis, ovarian dysfunction, prostatitis, and dozens of others. All these conditions have a common thread: the high likelihood of a systemic Candida infection. Symptoms of candidiasis are equally diverse. These symptoms include fatigue, mental fog, confusion, PMS, menstrual cramps, sugar cravings, especially during menses, chronic respiratory problems, digestive disorders, allergies, hives, heartburn, spastic colon, diarrhea, constipation, bloating, vaginitis, itching of the vagina, itchy skin, itching of the penis, prostate problems, chronic bladder problems, stuffy sinuses, ear infections, persistent bronchitis, itching of the ear canals and belly button plus dozens more. For a more detailed list of symptoms that an individual can test for see the Yeast Overload test in Nutritiontest.com. This is a for-pay testing system on the internet for a wide range of conditions and deficiencies.

Through such a test the individual can determine precisely his/her degree of infection plus the necessary therapy. See also the sections in this chapter, Mold, as well as Systemic fungus.

Treatment protocol

To treat this condition use a double-therapy approach: the oil under the tongue and the Oregacyn by mouth. Take 10 or more drops of the oil under the tongue three times daily. Also, take the Oregacyn, two capsules three times daily. For tough cases use the SuperStrength, 10 drops three times daily. High doses of the wild oregano may kill the natural bacteria. Replace these with the Health-Bac, one or two heaping teaspoons at night right before bedtime. Avoid the intake of refined sugar and processed foods as well as alcohol. Curtail the intake of sweets, white flour products, and white rice. Do not consume candy of any type. In candidiasis the hormone system is in disarray. By supporting both the thyroid gland and adrenals great improvement may be gained. For thyroid support take Thyroset, three capsules twice daily. In the case of adrenal weakness, which is particularly common in chronic candidiasis, also take the premium-grade royal jelly, that is the Royal Power, 4 capsules every morning. The combination of oregano therapy plus adrenal and thyroid support produces dependable results.

Ebola, dengue, or ebola-like syndromes (hemorrhagic fevers)

Ebola-like diseases should never be considered as being remote, that is only for the African villagers. Such diseases, that is hemorrhagic fevers, are striking even Westerners. During 2003 in the United States several people died from Ebola-like syndromes, but it was due to other types of viruses, like the dengue and SARS viruses. Dengue fever, a type of hemorrhagic fever similar to Ebola, infects hundreds of Americans yearly, most in the Deep Southwest.

Dengue is the most common type of hemorrhagic fever which afflicts Americans. It occurs primarily in the southwest, particularly in Texas, Arizona, southern California, and Hawaii. The mosquito which carries this fever, *Aedes aegypti*, appears to be adapting from its normally tropical habitat to more temperate regions. Currently, there is a massive epidemic in Indonesia, killing dozens of people daily. Yet, a type of hemorrhagic fever has developed in northern California. There, in a San Francisco Bay hospital several people died a most vile death—bleeding to death through their lungs, kidneys, and intestines. Deaths from a similar syndrome are also occurring in New York State. In the San Francisco outbreak local workers have correlated the deaths with a freakish trend: the performance by humans of sex acts with animals. The humans become infected with the animal viruses, which mutate, becoming potent human killers. The viruses are then spread by close contact, not necessarily sexual.

Treatment protocol

As a therapy to prevent internal bleeding take the crude red grape powder (i. e. Resvital), two or more teaspoons twice daily. Take also unprocessed natural vitamin C, that is Purely-C, three or more capsules several times daily. As a potent natural antiseptic take Oreganol oil, five or more drops under the tongue several times daily. In severe instances take it as often as every five minutes. Take also Oregacyn, two or more capsules several times daily. Oregacyn is hemostatic, which means it helps halt bleeding. For dire cases use the Oregacyn frequently, like a capsule or two every half hour, always with food or juice. Use the Germ-a-Clenz to decontaminate any suspect room or region. Spray it into the face to prevent the spread of contagion. Avoid spraying into eyes.

Recent evidence implicates mites in the transmission of hemorrhagic fevers. Spray the Germ-a-Clenz over the entire body. Also, spray all bedding or other potentially contaminated surfaces. Rub the oil into the skin, especially over the lymphatic points on the back of the wrists, along the thighs, and over the upper chest. After showering mist the Germ-a-Clenz all over the skin, avoiding direct contact with the genitals. Also, rub the Oreganol up and down the spine, especially after showering.

Encephalitis viruses

There are dozens of encephalitis viruses. Many of these viruses originate in animals. Humans are infected through the bites of blood-feeding insects, particularly mosquitoes and ticks as well as mites.

Encephalitis viruses infect a wide range of animals. Mice, rats, birds, and large mammals all carry these viruses. The viruses may cause fatal diseases in such animals, however, the primary danger is if they jump species. Perhaps most well known encephalitis viruses are the types which infect horses. Examples of these include the St. Louis encephalitis virus, Japanese equine encephalitis virus, and the West Nile virus. Horses are readily infected with these viruses through the bites of ticks and mosquitoes. The horses are further bitten by such insects, which then bite humans. These viruses are aggressive germs. They readily infect the nervous system, causing cell damage, even death. They are called neurotropic viruses, which means they are capable of invading nerve cells, feeding off them, and then destroying them. Humans are the final host, and horses are the intermediate one. This means that once humans are infected they are, in general, unable to transmit the infection to others. In other words, even if they are bitten by a mosquito and, then, that mosquito bites others, no transmission will occur.

Most of the encephalitis viruses are arboviruses. These viruses readily infect mammals and birds. Mosquitoes contract the virus from infected mammals, particularly rodents and birds. The infected mosquitoes or ticks then infect horses. After feeding on horses these arthropods attack humans, causing viral contamination. Such contamination may result in the full-fledged disease. Or, it may cause a subtle infection, which can either be self-limiting or result in chronic disease. Symptoms of infection by encephalitis viruses varies greatly from a mild illness with fever and aches to obvious neurological disease. However, common symptoms of the more serious type include fever with physical collapse, swelling of the lymph nodes, especially in the neck, rash, hemorrhaging, paralysis, and muscle weakness. The infection may be self-limiting, or it may lead to either meningitis or encephalitis, both of which are potentially fatal.

The virus enters the body through mosquito bites. The mouths, that is probiscus, of mosquitoes are teeming with it. From the skin it is carried into the blood, where it enters the internal organs and lymphatic tissue. The immune system attempts to destroy or inhibit it. However, frequently, the immune system is compromised and, thus, it fails to destroy the virus. Thus, it evades all defenses, multiplying in vast numbers. Ultimately, it enters the brain, where it further multiplies. The virus infects brain cells, where these organisms multiply by the trillions. In a few mere minutes the body may be fully overcome, well before the immune system can mount a defense. Each brain cell may contain untold millions of viruses, which systematically deplete it of all vitality. The pressure upon such cells is so great that they usually die, bursting to release the potentially deadly viruses.

Brain cells are irreplaceable. In nature they simply don't die. Viruses are highly destructive to such cells, infecting them and, ultimately, killing them. Yet, the encephalitis viruses specialize in attacking brain cells, and they do so with frightening efficiency. The extent of this destruction determines if the symptoms of encephalitis develop. Incredibly, a mild-to-minimal destruction may not cause the syndrome. Yet, this disease can be insidious. It may happen while the victim is virtually unawares: a mild headache, a stiff neck, a stiff back, a bit of a fever. Yet, this is a signal that the virus has invaded the brain and/or spinal cord, where it causes extensive damage. In other words, nerve cells begin dying. As the encephalitis progresses detritus, that is cellular waste, in fact, dead cellular matter from cells killed by the virus, is produced. This detritus is further attacked by the immune system, which aggravates the illness. The resulting inflammation stalls healing. Depending upon the degree of damage it may take months for the victim to recover, if ever.

The immune system responds vigorously to the attack. Antibodies against the virus are produced in vast quantities. These attack both the dying cells, the detritus, and the viruses, leading to further inflammation. Toxins and dead cells accumulate, disrupting the flow of blood and lymph. In fact, blood vessels in the brain may be obstructed by such material. The material then accumulates in the ventricles of the brain and, ultimately, the spinal fluid.

W. T. Hubbert, editor of the book, *Diseases Transmitted from Animals to Man*, describes how the antibody-virus combination is likely the cause of clogged blood vessels, which commonly develops in encephalitis. In fact, the arteries in the brain can be largely destroyed by such a process. This may lead to internal hemorrhaging, that is stroke. Or, it may cut off the flow of blood and, therefore, oxygen, which may also lead to brain damage as well as stroke.

Viruses are implicated in a variety of neurological diseases. These germs readily attack the brain, and infection need not be acute. A variety of chronic diseases may be caused by brain-attacking viruses, including multiple sclerosis, ALS, Parkinson's disease, and Alzheimer's disease. In multiple sclerosis a herpes virus is implicated, although, admittedly, several viruses may be involved. In ALS the main culprit appears to be an echovirus, although a variety of other germs have also been recently implicated, including chlamydia and rodent spirochetes. In Parkinson's and Alzheimer's the offending agent is unknown, although herpes, as well as encephalitis viruses, has been implicated. This is why encephalitis viruses are listed as a cause of pandemics: their role in the cause of chronic disease is significant. The fact is in the United States Alzheimer's and Parkinson's disease are true plagues. What's more, such diseases have developed in pockets, confirming an infectious origin. While in Alzheimer's disease a variety of viruses have been implicated, much of the evidence points to a relatively common one: the herpes virus. It is well known that the brains of Alzheimer's victims develop particular types of lesions, where the brain tissue is disrupted into messy tangles. These tangles contain a protein known as beta amyloid. Researchers at the University of California Irvine have discovered that this protein is essentially the same as the herpes simplex-1 virus, the same one which causes cold sores. These researchers created a sort of synthetic herpes, injecting it into brain cells. The result was that the brain cells were destroyed, that is disrupted into the typical tangles, just like in Alzheimer's disease.

Obviously, in this disease the brain cells are being attacked, although the exact germ(s) is unknown. Recently, in addition to herpes researchers have found a variety of germs within the brains of Alzheimer's victims, including herpes and chlamydia. It only makes sense that this would be a microbe. Viruses are one of the few types of microbes readily capable of penetrating the blood-brain barrier. It is well established that a wide range of neurological diseases are due to viruses. Bacteria can also penetrate the brain. For instance, syphilis causes an Alzheimer's-like syndrome. In fact, in some instances Alzheimer's may represent a type of chronic inherited syphilis of the brain. Recently, researchers have claimed to find a variety of other bacteria in Alzheimer's patients. These bacteria include chlamydia and a bacteria-like fungus known as actinomycetes. The latter is a tentacle-creating germ, which is highly invasive. The latest data shows that at least 90% of all Alzheimer's patients have active brain infection, largely by chlamydia.

Actinomycoses is a normal resident of the mouth. It may enter the brain through invasive medical procedures, particularly dentistry. It may eventually be proven that this germ plays a role in the destruction of brain cells so commonly seen in Alzheimer's disease. The organism resides in the mouth and readily infects diseased teeth. Obviously, anatomically, the teeth are exceptionally close to the brain. Thus, invasive dentistry may disseminate this infection, even driving the germs directly into the brain. In the 1950s dentists in Canada made such a finding: the brain is readily infected, that is through invasive dentistry. These dentists found in brain tissue dozens of types of germs, including a wide range of fungi, which had infected the brain through dental contamination. The source of this germ was contaminated teeth and/or instruments, and through invasive dentistry the infections were apparently driven directly into the brain.

It is interesting to note the connection between the introduction of vaccines and Alzheimer's disease. The latter was virtually unknown in this country until the mid-20th century, the very time in which vaccines were popularized. John Lear documents in his book, *Recombinant DNA*, that commercial vaccines are extensively contaminated with viruses, many of which are neurotropic. The latter means they have a specific ability to attack and infect brain or nerve cells. Among these is the notorious simian virus 40, which is a type of herpetic virus. In fact, this is a venereal-type virus transmitted sexually between monkeys. It is a kind of monkey VD. Medical sources indicate such contamination occurred primarily in vaccines made in the 1950s through 60s. Yet, the fact is any commercial vaccine is contaminated with either viruses or viral genetic material. Such vaccines are impossible to purify. Claims that they have been purged have now been refuted. Thus, even today's vaccines are contaminated.

The majority of these contaminants are of animal origin. Many of these viruses are aggressive pathogens, attacking and destroying human tissue, including the brain. These viruses usually cause a type of stealth infection, and, while acute infections do occur, they are less common. In other words, don't rule out vaccine-induced infections as a cause of a specific disease, including neurological disorders, just because there was no sudden post-vaccination reaction. The fact is hundreds of millions of North Americans are infected by vaccine-induced stealth viruses (see the Simian virus section).

There may be yet another major source for the Alzheimer's and Parkinson's epidemic: hormonal drugs. Recently, a study by *JAMA* concluded that women who take such drugs are more than twice as likely to develop Alzheimer's disease as non-users. While previous studies have documented an increased risk in estrogen users of heart disease and stroke, as well as breast cancer, the risk for dementia and Alzheimer's is far more considerable. This is seemingly the number one risk from taking such drugs. There must be a plausible explanation for such a dramatic increase in incidence. Estrogens alone fail to account for it.

A doubling of the risk is highly significant. Tens of millions of women take or have taken potent estrogenic drugs, either for post-menopausal hormonal support or for specific diseases. What's more, they have taken such drugs on the basis that their health would improve. Yet, the risk of taking such drugs is high, far greater than any potential benefits. One reason is the possibility of contamination. The majority of these drugs are animal derived. Specifically, they are extracted from the urine of pregnant horses. For instance, Premarin is made exclusively from pregnant mares' urine. The horses are artificially inseminated and 'farmed' just for this purpose. These relatively enormous animals produce vast amounts of a potent kind of estrogen, far too potent for human use, which is metabolized and excreted into the urine. The horses are forcibly impregnated; the estrogen produced is highly potent and is only applicable to this species. What's more, the type of estrogen which is excreted is not the ideal: it is a waste product. Plus, this urine is contaminated with a plethora of dangerous viruses, as well as other unknown germs, many of which are capable of attacking the nervous system, particularly the brain. Here is the critical issue: how can urine be sterilized, that is short of heating it to super-high temperatures? Drug companies harvest the estrogens, and to be effective such drugs must be active. Heating destroys the activity. Obviously, these companies are unable to sterilize the urine. The fact is urine contains trillions of microbes. It is a waste product, never fit for human consumption. Nor are any hormones secreted in it. It is contaminated with a variety of microbial components, including viruses, mycoplasmas, phages, molds, parasites, and bacteria, perhaps prions. Certainly, depending upon the type of feed given to these animals the prion content could be considerable. This is the only plausible cause for the increase in Alzheimer's disease, which occurs in those taking the drugs. It can't be from the estrogens alone; if such hormones were toxic, other organs would be damaged such as the liver and kidneys.

Remember, horses carry a wide range of neurologically active viruses, including the encephalitis viruses, which are excreted in the urine.

The only possibility is that the pills themselves are transmitting disease in the form of Alzheimer's disease-inducing germs or perhaps germ or viral genetic material, which creates a toxic reaction in the brain. Or, the urine is contaminated with prions, which would fully explain the high incidence of this disease in horse-urine estrogen users. Perhaps it is corrupted with submicroscopic bacteria such as mycoplasma. Or, possibly it contains fragments of viral and bacterial DNA or RNA, which, once digested and absorbed, induces inflammation and autoimmune reactions. Another possibility is that these drugs contain submicroscopic toxins—bacterial or mold toxins—which damage or destroy nerve and brain tissue. Yet, the most likely scenario is that such drugs are contaminated with a wide range of microbial particles or even live microbes themselves. The fact is horses are carriers of a wide range of viruses, which specialize in attacking the central nervous system. These are known as encephalitis viruses. A partial list of the viruses which may be found in horses' urine includes rabies, encephalitis, pox, relapsing fever, infectious anemia, and West Nile. When the estrogens are removed from the urine, certainly, this material is either contaminated with viruses or viral particles. Viruses are routinely excreted through the urine. Plus, the urine is contaminated with toxins produced by such microbes. How could such germs, germ components, and toxins be removed? The fact is such a technology fails to exist. Thus, it would be impossible to remove them completely. What's more, the agents used to sterilize such toxins, formaldehyde, aluminum salts, and mercurial compounds, are themselves toxic. Such components must ultimately cause disease. This may largely explain the increased risk in users of estrogen pills of brain disorders, neurological diseases, heart attacks, arterial diseases, cancer, and strokes. All the aforementioned have been connected to infections.

The fact that Alzheimer's disease is significantly more common in post-menopausal women than any other group is further proof of the connection. In North American women it is nearly 2.5 times more common in females than males. In English women it is nearly 4 times more common. What's more, it nearly always strikes Western women at 60 years or older. A high percentage of these women were hormone users. Furthermore, the incidence of this disease in non-Western women is virtually nil. Regarding the latter these are women who fail to take estrogen replacement drugs. For instance, in the villages of Greece and Turkey Alzheimer's among elderly women is virtually unknown, despite their reaching ages of up to 95 years or more. What is the only distinguishing factor? Certainly, this cannot be explained by the slightly higher longevity of women. Nor can it be explained by the difference in diet or climate. Turkish and Greek villagers, in fact, eat a considerable amount of processed food, especially refined sugar, white rice, and sweets. Rather, it is the fact that in the West hundreds of millions of women have for some 50 years been taking horse urine estrogens. It may also be related to another debacle: common vaccines. This is because vaccines introduce a wide range of germs, as well as germ DNA, which are capable of infecting the nervous system.

Drug makers have never provided proof of safety for animal estrogens. On the contrary drug company studies document a dangerous consequence: a significant increase in breast cancer. For decades it has been known that horse-urine estrogen can cause cancer. Thus, tens of thousands of lives have been lost unnecessarily, as well as untold misery caused, all to feed corporate profits. Furthermore, such estrogens have been fully confirmed to cause cancer. Their cancer-causing effects were well published prior to their introduction in the 1960s. Yet, the potential for microbial contamination had never been thoroughly assessed. Hundreds of researchers have attributed the cause of Alzheimer's to infection, the emphasis being viruses. This gives credence to the theory that, in fact, urine-derived drugs may be a major cause of this disease. The fact is urine is the body's means of excreting both toxins and microbes, including viruses. Thus, any derivative will be toxic. In other words, how can estrogen be purified when it is an excretory product? Therefore, anything which is derived from the urine is toxic. The fact is the pharmaceutical industry has perpetrated a global fraud upon the public. In my practice over a period of ten years I never once prescribed urine-derived estrogens. Yet, doctors freely prescribed, some even mandating, their use. Patients who may have been hesitant were often coerced into taking them. Yet, this was all for naught. According to the *New England Journal of Medicine* the routine intake of potent urine-derived estrogens offers "no...meaningful benefits" in any aspect of women's' lives. What a dire conclusion for those who took an agent that was supposed to benefit them. The fact is the public placed its trust in the estrogens as a health aid, not a killer. Is there anything produced by the pharmaceutical houses which can be trusted? Estrogenic drugs were one of the biggest selling drugs of all time. Untold millions of women faithfully took them. However, these drugs have been now proven to be the cause of a pandemic, an entire health disaster directly caused by the very agencies, the pharmaceutical houses, entrusted to aid and preserve human health. Women throughout the globe truly believed they were helping themselves by taking hormone replacement therapy, all the while contributing to their own demise. This is one of the greatest medical debacles of all time.

Treatment protocol

As a natural antiseptic to purge stealth germs and neurologically active viruses take oil of wild oregano (Oreganol P73), five or more drops under the tongue two or more times daily. For difficult situations take it aggressively, like five to ten drops every few minutes. Also, take Oregacyn, two capsules three or more times daily with food. Consume one or two raw organic egg yolks in a natural milk shake, for instance, the Nutri-Sense shake. Be sure the eggs are organic. In a blender add two egg yolks, three tablespoons Nutri-Sense, pine nuts/blanched almonds, or whole organic yogurt; add raw honey and fruit for taste and blend, adding water to desired thickness. Also, to ensure sterility (i.e. of the egg yolks) add a few drops of edible spice-based Oreganol to neutralize any potential microbes. Drink daily as a brain-nourishing shake. Drink also the Oreganol P73 Juice, one or two ounces twice daily. This water-soluble form of wild oregano crosses the blood-brain barrier to deliver its potency directly to the brain. Raw honey boosts immunity, while balancing digestion. Take a tablespoon twice daily. Also, eat large amounts of hot vegetables, particularly onions, radishes, garlic, and green onions. Make a juice from hot vegetables, using arugula, watercress, radishes, and green onions. Drink a cup or more daily. Also, take Neuroloft capsules, three or more capsules twice daily. This helps heal and reactivate the brain cells.

Flu

Practically, this is the most important infective cause of death to consider. The flu should not be taken lightly. It has a rather sordid history. Every year it kills on average some 30,000 to 36,000 Americans, primarily the elderly. However, no one is immune to its potentially devastating powers. Even the relatively healthy and fit could succumb to it. Yet, regarding its yearly devastation that is an incredibly high number, considering that the flu virus is not exceedingly tough. For instance, certain bacteria, such as staph and pseudomonas, as well as certain yeasts, such as candida, are far hardier.

The potency of the flu virus varies greatly. In pandemic years the number of deaths rises significantly. In an extreme year in North America alone up to 80,000 may die. Thousands more may be crippled by it, never fully recovering.

At any moment and in any year the flu may prove devastating. Without warning it could convert into an unrelenting international killer. This is what happened in 1918. What's more, it happened in numerous centuries prior. Since the late Middle Ages every century to date has been visited with a killer flu pandemic. Such flu strains struck rapidly and without warning, causing an international epidemic. What's more, humans lacked any immunity against such strains. The fact is the next one, that is the one which is expected to afflict modern civilization, is long overdue. If it is even remotely similar to the 1918 version, the world will endure utter pandemonium. Then, as many as 40 to 60 million died, some 1% of the global population. This would be virtually impossible to conceive of today. A comparable percentage of today's population would amount to some 100,000,000, an unfathomable number of souls. This would be absolute mayhem. Thus, reviewing the 1918 scenario aids in understanding the potential scope.

In 1918 the flu struck with a ferocity never before known. The attack was short-lived, some four months. The results were devastating. This was no ordinary flu. The virus seemed to prefer previously healthy individuals, particularly healthy men and women about 20 to 44 years of age. Servicemen were primary victims, as were healthy laborers. A person might even have failed to understand he/she was ill and, while seemingly in a normal condition would suddenly collapse, dying instantly. Others would die within two or three days, while enduring agonizing symptoms. People simply fell dead, without warning. What's more, they failed to die peacefully: they bled to death. The fact is the pandemic flu virus proved to be a hemorrhagic type, similar in its mechanism to Ebola. Upon autopsy physicians discovered a grisly fact: the virus attacked and destroyed the human organs, converting them into a blood soup. This was a true hemorrhagic virus, which kills through internal bleeding. Madeline Drexler, author of *Secret Agents: The Menace of Emerging Infections*, quotes one New York physician, who said "They're as blue as huckleberries and spitting blood." The blood loss was so severe, as Drexler describes, that people became blue: cyanotic. The blue discoloration "extended from the ears and spread all over the face."

It all began not as a natural epidemic but as a consequence of war. The virus broke out in the United States at a military camp. Here, soldiers were arriving in droves from Europe. The soldiers had experienced trench warfare and, thus, had developed a wide range of infectious diseases. They were immunocompromised due to their exposure to the elements, chemical gases, and vaccinations. The trenches, reeking of human debris, attracted rats, which, perhaps, like the hemorrhagic SARS virus, may have been the source for the germ.

The servicemen, who were heavily vaccinated, were an ideal medium for the spread of pandemic germs, particularly the flu. The fact is they were among the flu's primary victims. A greater number of U. S. servicemen died from this disease than from the war itself. Like SARS the 1918 flu became established at the end of winter: March. Even today the flu may peak in this month. In droves soldiers flocked to the base hospital complaining of fever and malaise. According to Drexler:

Within a month the virus had reached most American cities. American doughboys, jammed into troopships, ferried the germ to Europe. Yet, while it clearly represented a new round of the flu, this spring wave didn't set off any alarms. In June the Spanish wire service cabled Reuters in London: "A strange form of disease of epidemic character has appeared in Madrid...the epidemic is of a mild nature, no deaths having been reported." In so informing a world at war, Spain...inadvertently bestowed its name on the...infection. By July...(it) had spread around the world."

Thus, as the aforementioned demonstrates, rather than this being truly of Spanish origin it was, rather, an American flu of Chinese origin. It spread from the Americans through U.S. servicemen through the rest of the world. As expected, in the summer the virus went in remission. Flu viruses are highly vulnerable to heat, especially intense sunlight. However, there was a most unexpected consequence: a fall resurgence. The virus mutated, converting into a fulminant killer. No one was immune. Even the most powerful and healthy could succumb. The mutation turned the virus into a voracious killer, wiping out formerly healthy people in days, in fact, minutes. Highly contagious, it initially caused cold-like symptoms, which could spread nearly immediately. Due to the vigorous nature of the virus minor contact could spread the infection. The germ was fully airborne. The mere exposure to air in a closed area filled with humans was sufficient to initiate the infection. Symptoms included congestion, aches, backache, headache, fever, and pain in the eyes, head, and ears. Most people recovered. However, others developed violent illnesses. People simply collapsed and died.

Drexler's *Secret Agents*, perhaps the best book on the subject, gives the following description:

The microbe's target was not only the lining of...the respiratory tract, where flu usually takes up its residence, but also the tiny air sacs at the terminal branches of the respiratory system, deep in the lung—the alveoli, where oxygen and carbon dioxide are exchanged. Composed of hundreds of millions of these delicate air-filled structures, healthy lungs are light and buoyant, able to float in water. Lungs removed from the victims of the 1918 flu were hideously transformed: dense, heavy, the alveoli saturated with bloody fluid. Patients died by drowning. As rigor mortis set in, bloody froth streamed from their noses, staining their bed sheets.

On the radio during my interview with Bill Boshears of Cincinnati's WLW, a caller asked an important question: how can a more severe flu be distinguished from a less serious or more mild case? As noted previously with pandemic flu there is no distinguishing. It is unpredictable. It may strike suddenly. There is no single pattern of symptoms to expect, other than a single ominous signal: unusual bleeding tendencies. If a person begins to bleed suddenly from the nose or ears or begins spitting up blood, this is a dire sign. It is a warning that the body is being viciously attacked: by a hemorrhagic virus. It may be flu or it may be SARS or SARS-like. Regardless of the cause if the condition is neglected, that is if there is a failure to prescribe the appropriate treatment, serious consequences, including organ failure and/or death, may result. Thus, it is important to never take chances and, in fact, to know precisely what to do. This is what this section will achieve. There is no reason to succumb. Through the information in this book anyone can halt the killer flu. Thus, regardless of what is happening throughout the world—even utter death and devastation—anyone who applies the information in this book can essentially immunize the self. Thus, as long as these methods are adhered to rigorously—that is the regular intake of potent, wild spice extracts, particularly Oregacyn—there is no fear of death from the flu or for that matter any other form of contagion.

Regarding the flu and its potential for human devastation people are often apathetic. Even if millions are being harmed or killed, usually, people find no need to take action, that is unless they themselves are suffering from it. In *Secret Agents* Drexler confirms this. She says "The most dangerous misconception about flu is that it is nothing more than a bad cold." The fact is this illness can strike suddenly and can harm or even kill a perfectly healthy individual. This is precisely what happened during the 1918 epidemic. It is also what will happen in the future. Those who prepare may well save their lives, while many others who fail to prepare will likely succumb.

The key with the flu is to either prevent it or properly treat it, that is to minimize damage. This is because this illness is curable, even in its pandemic form. This is true if the individual knows exactly what to take and how much to take. The flu virus is readily destroyed by spice extracts, particularly oil of wild oregano and even to a greater degree, the multiple spice capsules, Oregacyn. Both the oregano oil and the Oregacyn are proven germ killers. Using a special blend of wild oregano (P73 Oreganol) researchers killed both the flu virus and coronavirus, the agent thought responsible for SARS. The P73 was tested against the toughest flu virus known: influenza A. The Oreganol was highly active against the viruses, killing some 99.9% within a mere 20 minutes. The Oregacyn proved even more powerful; it killed 100% of all viruses within 20 minutes. Thus, for life-threatening infections Oregacyn is the most potent. The fact is it obliterated all traces of both the coronavirus and influenza A, the cause of the most recent flu pandemic. This is not merely test tube research. The fact is the Oreganol and Oregacyn have been proven to kill viruses, as well as bacteria, in human tissue. No drug could ever achieve such results. Thus, the Oregacyn is more powerful than any pharmaceutical agent, that is in eradicating the common cold as well as flu. When taken, people usually notice a major impact upon respiratory symptoms. For certain it significantly reduces the duration of any respiratory illness. What's more, regarding sinus-related symptoms it has major impact, rapidly drying up and/or opening up the sinuses. What's more, it significantly reduces the typical agonizing symptoms of the flu: fever, chills, and aches. With Oregacyn there is no need to get violently ill. It blocks the development of such a severity.

In North America influenza is a major cause of disability as well as death. Untreated, it may precipitate a decline in immunity, which is potentially fatal. With a damaged immune system bacterial infection may develop. This may lead to bacterial bronchitis and, ultimately, bacterial pneumonia, which is fatal. Yet, this is largely unnecessary. All could be prevented. This is because the flu virus, as well as various noxious bacteria, readily succumb to spice extracts, particularly the Oregacyn. What's more, infection can be largely prevented by the regular intake of such substances.

Treatment protocol

Take oil of wild oregano, that is the P73 blend, 3 to 5 drops under the tongue as often as possible, even every few minutes, if necessary. It may be necessary to take mega-doses, 10 or more drops at a time. This can be repeated several times daily, even as often as every few minutes. Rub the oil on lymphatic spots such as the spots on the feet, hands, and upper chest. Also, do a spinal rub, vigorously rubbing the oil up and down the spinal column. Do this twice daily. Take also Oregacyn, 2 caps every four hours with food or juice. For severe cases take it every hour or even every half hour, always with food or juice. It may be taken on an empty stomach but only after the body becomes adjusted to it. For children add the oil or a pinch or two of the Oregacyn to raw honey. Take as often as needed. As it becomes readily tolerated increase the dose, a half capsule at a time.

Raw Mediterranean honeys, for instance, wild oregano or thistle honeys, are the ideal energy tonics to consume. Take one or more tablespoonsful several times daily. This is also invaluable for intestinal flu, particularly diarrhea. The intake of solid foods should be restricted. Avoid heavy foods, eating primarily fruit or clear broth soups. What's more, avoid the intake of meat, pork, and milk products as well as rich sauces. Strictly curtail the intake of sugar, chocolate, and alcohol. If you smoke, quit.

While dietary changes are important—it takes the burden off the immune system to eliminate noxious or chemically infested foods—it is only natural medicine that can effectively defend against the flu. It is possible to ward off this illness, as well as reverse it, with such medicines. The individual must take advantage of the most powerful natural medicines of all: spice extracts. This is because such extracts have been proven to kill the cold/flu viruses. In summary the flu defense kit should contain:

- wild oregano oil from the edible spice only (P73 Oreganol)

- the multiple wild spice capsules capable of destroying the flu and corona (i.e. cold) viruses, that is Oregacyn dry capsules

- high grade raw wild mountain honey, preferably the wild oregano honey (only available mail-order, 1-800-243-5242)

- Oreganol P73 Juice (optional) to halt any neurological components and to provide strength, especially for the elderly.

- Oregacyn oil, a cinnamon, sage, and oregano oil blend which, under the tongue, has a more pleasant taste than Oreganol. This is the ideal oil to use under the tongue for children: it may also be taken as a gelcap, which is small and, therefore, easy to swallow. Such an approach will defeat even the worst case of the flu, even in a severely weakened individual. The secret is to take if necessary huge doses, since the aforementioned are non-toxic. There is no medical reason to avoid taking the protocol except, perhaps, regarding the honey. Diabetics might prove intolerant of it, although, of all honeys the oregano type is the most well tolerated. A lesser protocol may be followed, that is merely the oil and the Oregacyn. Yet, for optimal results the entire protocol must be followed.

Yet, in the event of a pandemic modest doses may prove insufficient. It may be necessary to take enormous doses. With the oil a dropperful every ten or twenty minutes may be required. Remember, there may be untold trillions of viruses in the body. A major effort is required to kill them. With the Oregacyn two to four capsules every half hour or hour may be required. Regarding the juice it must be sipped on often; as much as a bottle daily. Honey may also be taken in large amounts, as much as four ounces daily.

There are other home remedies for the flu, which offer a certain degree of protection. These home remedies include garlic, onion, cinnamon sticks, cloves, ginger, and propolis. In particular, propolis extracts may prove invaluable. A powerful antiviral agent, it may be necessary to add propolis to any antiviral regimen. An emulsified Oil of Propolis in an oregano oil base is available (only by mail-order, 800-243-5242). Ginger is both a germicide and an anti-inflammatory agent. Thus, it may prove helpful in controlling many of the symptoms of flu, including muscle and joint aches, headache, back pain, and fever. Garlic and onion broth, combined with beef or chicken stock, is the ideal food to consume during the flu. Here is a recipe for an anti-flu garlicky chicken soup:

- 1/2 organic chicken, whole, with skin on (or) 1/2 to 1 pound beef soup bones
- 12 cloves garlic, minced

- 3 yellow onions, medium to large, chopped
- 3 bay leaves
- 2 teaspoons Hungarian paprika (optional)
- 2 teaspoons crude sea salt
- 3 drops Oreganol oil of wild oregano (or 2 tablespoons dried wild oregano from wild oregano bunches, not from spice shaker)
- bay leaves
- 1/3 to 1/2 head fresh organic broccoli, cut into medium to small pieces
- 8 fresh Brussels sprouts, sliced
- 1/3 to 1/2 head fresh organic cauliflower, broken into small pieces
- 1 large fresh red sweet pepper, cored, seeded, and chopped
- 1/2 cup fresh parsley, minced
- a few capsules of Purely-C and Resvital (to add at the end of cooking)

Wash chicken thoroughly. Rub a few drops of Oreganol on the carcass. In a large pot place chicken in water and boil for 20 to 30 minutes. If desired, skim off top layer of fluid. Add garlic, dried oregano, bay leaves, onions, garlic, and salt; continue cooking over reduced heat. Add vegetables, except parsley, which is added at the end of cooking. If using Oreganol, add this at the end. Also, at the end of cooking top with contents of a capsule of Purely-C and/or Resvital.

Note the emphasis on cruciferous vegetables. This is because these types of vegetables contain antibiotic-like substances. During the winter for ideal results eat a bowl of this soup regularly. In fact, this is a type of immune-boosting soup, loaded with natural antibiotics, sulfur compounds, and flavonoids. The broccoli, red sweet pepper, Brussels sprouts, and cauliflower provide vitamin C, that is if it is not boiled off. There is also a significant amount of vitamin C in the Purely-C and Resvital. Plus, recent evidence demonstrates that of all vegetables the cruciferous group, that is broccoli, cauliflower, cabbage, Brussels sprouts, kale, and others, offers the strongest immune support.

Citrus fruit is also invaluable, the fresher the better. Also, the pulp should be consumed. During the flu months be sure to consume fresh citrus fruit on a regular basis.

Bird flu

Flu viruses routinely infect birds. In fact wild birds naturally harbor such viruses. Yet, flu viruses usually fail to kill the birds. Rather, these animals act as carriers, in fact, reservoirs.

Under certain conditions such viruses can mutate, becoming potent killers. This is particularly true of bird viruses in Asia, that is the viruses infecting domestic birds. Here, a variety of farm animals live in close proximity, notably ducks, chickens, geese, and pigs. The pigs and chickens eat the feces of various animals, including ducks. The viruses are shed in the feces but are normally only mildly infective. Yet, it is the consumption of the infected feces that is largely responsible for the outbreaks. Chickens are the main victims. They are highly vulnerable to respiratory viruses. So are children, who are the primary human victims. Chickens eat the feces which are contaminated by this virus, allowing this aggressive virus to reproduce in their internal organs. From here it infects their lungs and is shed both in their secretions and feces. The virus is also disseminated into the air, both from dried droppings and via respiratory secretions. People contract it through contact with chicken feces, barn areas, perhaps the meat itself or eggs. What's more, it is airborne, and this is why it attacks and kills so suddenly.

Rarely, human diseases have been associated with birds, particularly ducks and chickens. Pigeons, as well as pet birds, may transmit various germs to humans, particularly certain fungi as well as the avian bacterial disease, psittacosis. Yet, the most dangerous are flu viruses, which have the ability to transfer to humans. Direct transfer is difficult. An intermediate is necessary. Hogs serve this function. Avian, that is bird viruses have become a major health threat. In fact, since 1997 a number of deaths have occurred in humans from such viruses, primarily in Hong Kong. In 1997 the deaths of several children and adults from such viruses, in this case, apparently, due to direct transfer from poultry to humans, led to the destruction of much of Hong Kong's poultry population.

A similar flu developed in February 1957, also originating in birds. Dead birds, including commercial poultry, were the first sign, just as is occurring today. Within six months the flu struck the United States, ultimately causing 70,000 deaths. This flu originated in poultry and pigs, and the same can be expected today. What's more, since it became established it simply won't disappear. The fact is it may cause a type of chronic infection, which may occasionally become reestablished. The current strain, H5N1, is some 50 years old. Obviously, it has established itself as a potentially constant threat.

The bird flu is an aggressive killer. Direct contact with infected birds can rapidly result in fatality. This is a hemorrhagic disease, which leads to the destruction of red, as well as white, blood cells, causing people to bleed to death. Plus, there is no immunity against it, nor any vaccine. These bird viruses may be closely associated with swine viruses, the latter being the primary source for human flu epidemics. Birds may develop the infection from infected pigs, since they are closely associated with it. The infection always arises in Asia, where pigs, fowl, and humans live in close proximity.

Recently, an ominous circumstance developed. In 2004 the bird flu resurfaced, killing within days millions of chickens. Simultaneously, it flipped to humans: suddenly, some 30 people were infected, most of whom died. The fact is in the early evolution of this disease the fatality rate is truly frightening: some 70%. This means that if ten people become infected, incredibly, only three will survive. These are the statistics provided by the WHO. What if this virus enters the general population? The results could be catastrophic. Normally, bird viruses have a difficult time crossing into other species, particularly humans. The virus cannot adapt to humans, that is without great difficulty. However, it can adapt readily within pigs. In fact, pigs act as the the genetic "mixing vessel", allowing the virus to genetically convert to a more virulent form. Then, it becomes a combination virus: part bird and swine. What's more, since pigs are in close proximity with humans, especially in Southeast Asia and China, the development of a human mutation is assured. Humans can, in fact, pass their varieties to pigs. Again, pigs act as a genetic mixing medium, blending the genes from all species, ultimately creating a highly invasive, in fact, deadly, agent. This is the source of the flu pandemics, which have ravaged humanity. Birds, including poultry, play a relatively minor role. It is the hogs which are the source of the deadly agents, which readily infect humans and which quickly adapt to human cells. W. T. Hubbert makes this clear in *Diseases Transmitted from Animals to Man*. He documents how it was swine which harbored and spread the 1918 killer flu. The swine virus infected uncountable masses of people, perhaps through contaminated meat, as well as direct contact with humans, perpetuating the epidemic. Soldiers were the primary victims. Interestingly, salt pork and canned pork products were major components of the military diet. Michael Oldstone, in his book, *Viruses, Plagues, and History*, demonstrates the connection:

Both avian (bird) and human influenza viruses can replicate in pigs, and genetic combinations between them can be demonstrated experimentally. A likely scenario for such an antigenic shift in nature occurs when the prevailing human strain of influenza A virus and an avian influenza virus concurrently infect a pig, which serves as a mixing vessel. Reassortants containing genes derived mainly from the human virus but with (a gene) from the avian source are able to infect humans and initiate a new pandemic. In rural Southeast Asia, the most densely populated area of the world, hundreds of millions of people live and work in close contact with domesticated pigs and ducks. This is the likely reason for the influenza pandemics.

Thus, when a person contracts influenza, he/she is, in fact, suffering from a germ of porcine origin from filth-generating hogs. What's more, this hog-derived germ is more fatal in humans than in the animal of origin. Consider the odor from a hog farm: during a flu infection that is the kind of filth which is attacking the body. It is a kind of filth capable of hurting the body: of killing it outright.

Be wary of the flu. It is far from a mild illness. Now (January 2004) doctors in Asia are faced with frightening consequences. It was Veronica Chan, M.D., chairman of the University of Philippine's College of Medicine, who made clear the dire reality. She said, "There is no protection from that new (bird-pig) virus, so it's going to cause a big epidemic." What's more, ominously, she made it clear that "We should worry. It kills, it kills." This is an attempt to give the West a warning, directly from the "front lines." The question is what is she seeing in Asia that the news media is failing to report? Dr. Chan is well aware that this is a violent killer, destroying peoples' internal organs, in fact, causing people to die by bleeding to death. If her words are regarded as accurate, this could be the global killer that has long been predicted, and it will begin killing immediately. The fact is this germ is so contagious that within days millions of chickens died. Millions of others have been culled. Within weeks it spread to some twelve countries, including the United States.

Yet, it is not the bird flu that is of the greatest concern. It is the mutation of such a flu virus within pigs, which has adapted to human tissue. The pigs usually survive. So, will the epidemic. The fact is when the human variation develops, fully brewed with proper genetics within pig's blood, this will be a killer beyond comprehension. Yet, the media in general makes light of it, claiming it has not been proven to spread from human to human. This is mere disinformation. Any contagion will eventually spread in such a manner, that is by direct contact with the infected individuals. All that is necessary is for the virus to reconstruct within pigs, which is already occurring. Pigs eat poultry/duck feces. In Asia these animals are relied upon as farmyard garbage cleaners. The pigs convert the ingested viruses into a porcine-poultry strain. Then, since these animals are in direct contact with humans, the germs from the humans themselves may be built into the virus. Now, the virus can readily attack humans. It develops the ability, genetically, to directly infect human cells, and the addition of genes from both poultry and pigs makes it highly vigorous. What's more, such a diverse structure makes it virtually impossible for the immune system to destroy it. It becomes a stealth virus which directly infects human cells, and there will be no immune response. No fever, chills, aches: in other words, without warning. The fact is such a germ can fully evade the immune system and directly infect human cells, even the white blood cells themselves. It becomes a monstrous virus, destroying all cells in its path. The fact is such a virus is a hemorrhagic virus, meaning it kills by causing people to bleed to death.

Without protection there is little hope for a cure. There is no medical therapy for such an infection. Only natural medicines, which directly destroy the virus, offer hope. Mere stimulation of the immune system, that is from agents such as Echinacea, elderberry, and goldenseal, while somewhat helpful, is insufficient. The germ must be rapidly destroyed. This is because it is highly fatal, and death can readily occur. What's more, dangerous symptoms can rapidly develop, which destabilizes health. Before a person can react he/she becomes violently ill. Frightened to death, the individual rushes to the doctor. Upon hospitalization there is no hope for a cure: only the Grace of Almighty God can be leaned upon. Thus, the virus must be destroyed through the powers of natural cures capable of outright killing viruses, since it is these substances alone which will save lives, that is if the bird flu virus converts to a human type.

Vigilance is necessary. During this risky time travel to the Orient should be curtailed. If you must travel, be sure to take a considerable supply of germicidal supplements, particularly the Oreganol and Oregacyn. Also, spray the air frequently with the spice extract Germ-a-Clenz. Take a natural bacterial supplement that does not require refrigeration such as Health-Bac (North American Herb & Spice). This will ensure the most reliable protection against killer germs.

Treatment protocol

Oregacyn or Oregacillin (i.e.the doctor's brand) multiple spice extract is the key supplement to take in order to destroy this infection. Take as much as is necessary to eliminate the infection. The dosage may vary, for instance, three capsules three times daily to as much as three capsules every half hour. Take with food, juice, or plenty of water. Oreganol oil of wild oregano: 10 to 20 drops under the tongue as often as possible, even every five minutes. In tough cases, particularly the bird flu, always use the SuperStrength. Take it as often as every few minutes, ideally under the tongue. Never be afraid of taking too much. The Oreganol P73 Juice is also invaluable for strength and stamina, as well as for reversing any neurological components. Take an ounce or more three times daily of Royal Oil unprocessed royal jelly: for strength and stamina, a squirt as often as possible. An easier way to take this is by capsule, that is the Royal Power high potency royal jelly. Take four capsules every morning. Take Wild Oregano or Thistle Honey: a tablespoon as often as possible. Eat as much wild raw honey as possible. Avoid eating large amounts of solid foods. During flu crisis eat lightly. For energy rely upon the raw honey and Royal Oil. Purely-C is a source of naturally occurring vitamin C: take 2 or more capsules several times daily.

Certain foods are protective, in fact, strength-producing. Such foods include organic meat broth soups, dark green leafy vegetables, papaya plus its seeds, hard kiwi fruit, fresh citrus fruit, grapefruit juice, tomato juice, garlic, onion, radishes, raw milk yogurt, wild berries, and raw honey. Avoid the consumption of heavy foods of all types, creamed soups, sweets, refined sugar, chocolate, tea, artificially sweetened beverages/food, deep fried food, nitrated meats, margarine, commercial milk products, cheese, and refined vegetable oils. Above all, remember it is only the Oregacyn P73 which obliterated cold/flu viruses in the test tube, killing all viruses within 20 minutes. This is a critical finding, that the viruses can be killed so rapidly. Thus, in the event of a new wave of a killer epidemic, including the vicious bird/porcine flu, the regular use of such a substance will definitely save lives. In case you are the victim take the Oregacyn, as well as the oil, vigorously. Your life will depend upon it.

There is another method to consider: intranasal use of Oreganol. This spice oil can be safely administered within the nasal canal. There is a special technique to do this. This is where the viruses congregate. They must be eliminated from this region in order to achieve a rapid cure. Simply saturate a

Q-Tip with the oil and slide up the nose along the inner nasal membrane. Allow contact as long as possible. Be careful to avoid contact with the sensitive outer membranes.

Hepatitis (A, B, and C)

This is an epidemic of vast proportions. It is due to a virus which aggressively attacks the liver. The hepatitis virus has a predisposition for liver cells. It lives in these cells, reproducing freely. From the liver tens of billions of such viruses are seeded in the blood. In fact, these viruses can be measured in the blood: by the tens of millions per milliliter. No wonder individuals with this disease are so violently sick, unable to maintain their health, barely holding on for survival.

All hepatitis viruses belong to the herpes family. Hepatitis C is a particularly aggressive agent. It viciously overpowers liver cells, conquering their genetic machinery. The virus induces the cells to produce their own genetic components, ultimately wearing them out and causing their deaths. For the liver to recover the virus must be destroyed. The fact is if the virus is allowed to continue to infect with impunity it not only destroys liver cells but also induces a dire consequence: liver cancer.

Hepatitis A is associated mainly with contamination by feces. This is the major type which causes food-related outbreaks. In the United States, September and November 2003, two enormous outbreaks of this infection occurred: all from eating restaurant food. The source was contaminated green onions, which were obviously unwashed or poorly washed. For one restaurant alone some 500 cases have been traced, including three deaths. All were patrons of a Chi-Chi's restaurant in Pennsylvania. In Atlanta a similar outbreak occurred, again tied to green onions: 12 restaurants were implicated. Yet, ultimately, it is not the restaurant: it is the grower. Apparently, these were imported green onions, grown in a region where human sludge is used as a fertilizer. Such sludge is extensively contaminated with highly toxic species of hepatitis as well as bacteria, parasites, and fungi. Unless such food is vigorously cleansed infection is inevitable. Even with thorough cleaning there is no guarantee of protection. Recent investigations found that sprouts grown on contaminated soil, regardless of how well they are washed, remain contaminated, the germs being absorbed within the shoots. Apparently, the toxic components, even the bacteria, are absorbed through the shoots and cannot be washed out. This demonstrates the value of the Oreganol as a food additive. If eating sprouts, add a few drops to the food/salad to ensure safety. Or, cut the sprouts from the base, and soak in a solution of water and a few drops of the Oreganol. The same can be done with any salad vegetables.

In the United States today there are at least six viruses known to cause liver disease. The hepatitis C viral (HCV) infection is the most common blood-borne viral infection. The prevalence of HCV is estimated at 1.8% of the American population (4.5 million people), of whom 2.7 million are chronically infected.

The government-approved treatment of hepatitis C is based upon combination therapy with interferon Alfa, a substance which mimics the natural immune response, and the antiviral drug, Ribavirin. This therapy produces results in about 50% of patients. However, the side effects are so dire that many people are rendered physically incompetent. Because of this people are resorting to a natural approach to manage or cure hepatitis. Numerous herbs, such as milk thistle, licorice root, ginseng and dandelion leaf, have an effect on the disease, with minor or even sustained improvement in liver enzymes and even a reduction in viral levels. Yet, a sustained cure has not been forthcoming. Now this has changed. Oregacyn, along with the oil of wild oregano, has been shown in a human trial to essentially reverse this disease. This pilot study, using Oregacyn P73 Liver Formula and Oreganol P73, was begun in May 2003. Oregacyn P73 Liver Formula is a proprietary blend of spice extracts with an Oreganol P73 base. This clinical trial in patients with hepatitis C demonstrated that Oreganol P73 and Oregacyn P73 Liver Formula possess direct antiviral activity against the hepatitis C virus. The initial results show that 80% of patients had a decrease in their HCV RNA (i.e. the genetic marker for active herpes viruses in the blood) titers, some showing a significant reduction in viral levels. This study is ongoing, with additional patients being enrolled. With the obvious benefits associated with the Oregacyn P73 Liver Formula and the Oreganol P73 in treating Hepatitis C there is no reason to look any further. After all, a safe, effective 100% wild spice extract without side effects is far superior to the potentially dangerous drugs. The fact is the combination of the Oreganol P73, which is taken sublingually, plus the LivaClenz has produced more superior results than any other previous medical therapy. This is without any serious side effects. What's more, in the majority of patients a noticeable reduction in liver enzymes has occurred, which is a sign that the natural therapy is completely non-toxic and, in fact, is causing a healing of damaged liver cells.

For more information on the hepatitis C study or to enroll in it contact a health resource specialist at 1-800-243-5242 or visit www.oreganol.com.

Treatment protocol

Hepatitis is tough to kill. Yet, while there are no drugs proven to kill it, spice extracts readily destroy it. A recent clinical trial has, in fact, proven that certain combinations of spice oils kill this virus, while healing liver tissue. What a side effect: positive benefits to the liver, while the virus is killed. This is the consequence of nature, in fact, the divine being. Only such a being could design such a medicine: powerful enough to kill the virus, while preserving, in fact, enhancing, organ function. Katherine Kirk, a veteran of hepatitis C infection, is an excellent example. As a result of the regular use of the spice oil, SuperStrength Oreganol, her viral levels plummeted from some 5,500,000 viral parts per milliliter, that is of blood, to a mere 450. This while her liver enzymes were normalized from some 400 to 20. It is a stupendous result, unheard of in the medical annals. This is the consequence of taking advantage of the powers of nature, which any hepatitis C victim can gain. The synthetics are valueless, in fact, counterproductive. Nature's medicines are curative, that is the medicines created by the Highest Power: God almighty. The natural medicine is an exact fit for the body, not only reversing the disease but also healing all tissues. To treat this condition take SuperStrength Oil of Oreganol, 20 drops under the tongue twice daily. Also, take the specially designed and researched LivaClenz, 2 to 3 capsules three times daily with meals. As a liver purge take also the GreensFlush, made from unprocessed raw green vegetables from the northern wilderness, 40 to 80 drops twice daily, ideally in an ounce of extra virgin olive oil.

Lyme

Lyme disease and its variants are caused by germs originating from rodents. The ticks feed on the rodents and then attach to humans. The rodent-derived germs are then directly injected into human blood.

Lyme disease was first recognized in 1975, due to an outbreak of a bizarre syndrome in Old Lyme, Connecticut. The syndrome was characterized by a severe type of arthritis, afflicting primarily children. Yet, Lyme is far from new. A similar disease was known in Europe. Here, the disease was called erythema migrans, the latter term indicating a traveling rash. Doctors were confused. What they regarded as a harmless skin disorder, in fact, often resulted in debilitating neurological disorders, even stroke. Certainly, the sudden epidemic nature of the infection is suspicious. Yet, even in the United States isolated cases have occurred, which were assuredly Lyme. As described by Arno Karlen in his book, *Man and Microbes,* isolated cases of this disease were reported in Long Island, New York, long before the Connecticut outbreak.

Ticks are blood-suckers. Thus, they carry a wide range of germs—whatever is in the blood. Perhaps most dangerous are the spirochetes, which are corkscrew-like bacteria. These bacteria are highly invasive and specialize in invading the central nervous system, that is the brain and spinal cord. *Borrelia burgdoferi*, a spirochete, is regarded as the cause of Lyme. Yet, it is implausible that this disease is caused only by one germ. Ticks are infested with hundreds, perhaps thousands, of species of germs. All are injected as a result of tick bites. Thus, tick bites cause a generalized sepsis, not a singular infection. For instance, it has only recently been determined that people with Lyme disease may also be infected by a parasite, the disease being known as babesiosis. The organism responsible for this disease is rather large and is known as a trophozoite, a true intracellular parasite similar to the organism which causes malaria. Like the malarial organism this parasite invades the red blood cells. Extreme exhaustion is one of the major symptoms of this infection. Other symptoms/signs of this infection include fevers, which are cyclical, drenching night sweats, joint pain, headache, abdominal pain, dark-colored urine, lowered white blood cell count, and elevated liver enzyme levels. Yet a third major pathogen has been recognized: *Ehrlichia chaffeenis*, the cause of ehrlichiosis. This germ causes a highly aggressive infection that has a high fatality rate: some 10 to 15%. Infection by this bacteria is regarded as a medical emergency. It is thought to be a canine bacteria, which ticks contract from feeding on dogs. The germ could also arise from rodents, which ticks also feed on. Yet, the fact is virtually anyone with a tick bite could contract all three infections simultaneously. Soon, new tick-borne pathogens will be found and new diseases will be named, again with bizarre names derived from either the site of discovery or the discoverer's' names.

Yet, spirochetes play a predominant role in the progression of Lyme. Here, these organisms invade the internal organs, particularly the brain and spinal cord, where they attack the cells. In nerve cells these spirochetes apparently feed off the cell membrane: the myelin sheath. Thus, they essentially strip this sheath from the cells, leading to severe damage, a condition known as demyelination. This process also occurs in multiple sclerosis. Thus, many cases of multiple sclerosis may, in fact, be undiagnosed Lyme. The fact is Lyme is an epidemic beyond comprehension. Potentially millions of North Americans suffer from this infection. Remember, the tick is only the carrier. The cause is rodent, as well as canine, derived germs.

Rodent-derived germs cause severe disease. They are stealth pathogens, which readily evade the immune system. These forms are known as pleomorphs. The suffix "morph" is descriptive. This is because such germs convert into various forms to evade immune detection.

The symptoms of Lyme disease are often vague. Unless there is a high degree of suspicion physicians often miss the diagnosis. In fact, a wide variety of chronic ailments may be due to Lyme. These include chronic arthritis, chronic fatigue syndrome, fibromyalgia, ankylosing spondylitis, bursitis, meningitis, Bell's palsy, heart disease, heart rhythm disturbances, hepatitis, encephalitis, and even dementia. Thus, incredibly, Alzheimer's-like presentations may, in fact, be undiagnosed Lyme.

Treatment protocol

The Lyme spirochetes burrow into brain and nerve tissue. Due to its ability to cross the blood-brain barrier the Oreganol P73 Juice is crucial: drink at least an ounce twice daily. Hold the juice in the mouth as long as possible before swallowing. To make it more palatable it may be added to tomato or V-8 juice or, perhaps, fresh-squeezed vegetable juice. Also, take the potent antiseptic spice pill Oregacyn, two capsules twice daily. Take also the Oreganol oil of wild oregano under the tongue, 10 or more drops three or more times daily. For fatigue and exhaustion take the unprocessed royal jelly, that is the Royal Power, four to six capsules every morning before breakfast. Also, as an additional aromatic essence take the Rosemary Essence, two ounces twice daily in hot water. This rosemary essence also crosses the blood-brain barrier. A topical therapy can also be applied. Simply rub the spine up and down with the Oreganol. The SuperStrength is the preferable type for this purpose. This will drive the medicine into the spinal tissues, where the actions are most needed. The oil may also be rubbed up and down the thighs. For lymphatic drainage an upward rubbing motion is preferable.

The Lyme bacteria is difficult to kill. In order to do so a prolonged therapy is required. At least a six month course of therapy is advisable.

Mad cow (i.e. Creutzfeldt-Jakob disease)

Mad cow is a misleading term. The afflicted cow is far from mad. Rather, it is writhing in agonizing pain. It is utterly distressed, since it is dying a brutal, unmerciful death: all man-induced. It might act aggressively, but only because it is in such dire agony. In other words, it moves about unpredictably, because it is writhing in pain and because it is suffering from significant brain damage. Thus, any aggressive behavior is due to severe damage to the brain and spinal cord, not any inherent madness.

Creutzfeldt-Jakob disease (CJD) is a fatal degenerative disease of the brain and spinal cord, that is the central nervous system. It primarily attacks the elderly, but, increasingly, younger people are falling victim: teenagers and 30 to 40 year olds.

The signs and symptoms of CJD are far from dependable. A significant variance can occur. However, memory loss is a common symptom, as are behavioral changes. The behavior may be bizarre—the person may become even agitated and/or hostile. There may be headaches and the unusual symptom of distortions in the appearance of objects. As the disease progresses the person may suffer delusions and even hallucinations. Confusion may develop, similar to Alzheimer's disease. Spasticity of the body strikes, like contortions, and there may even develop convulsions, even seizures. Then, problems with normal walking and balance occur—the victims lose normal coordination, in other words, the ability to walk is visibly disturbed. Normal speech is also disturbed; speech is garbled, in other words, there is slurred speech, largely due to the loss of muscle control, the result of nerve damage. Ultimately, the muscles atrophy, which can be one sided or systemic, followed by severe spasticity and rigidity. With loss of body control the tissues are greatly weakened. Infection strikes, and the individual rapidly succumbs, usually to pneumonia. This is the typical evolution of this disease. Yet, there are a number of variations of this disease, the so-called CJD variants. All are due to severe infections and/or toxicity within brain tissue.

In this condition the brain is extensively traumatized. At first brain cells grow excessively, but, ultimately, they are killed. Nerve cells eventually disappear, being replaced by mere shells. There is no inflammation: just cell death. The cells revert from healthy functional entities to as if balloons. This is known as balloon degeneration. This degeneration is the origin of the term spongioform. Thus, the cell death occurs in pockets, in fact, holes. In other words, the CJD agent aggressively destroys brain tissue, which is why neurological symptoms develop. The spinal cord is also destroyed, manifested by cellular swelling and also loss of cells. Ultimately, the entire spinal cord degenerates.

This disease is readily transmitted. The easiest way to contract it is through direct invasion, where the agent gains entrance through the skin: in other words, inoculation. Surgery is another route. So is anesthesia. It may also be contracted through blood transfusions, and there are a few cases in the United States which are confirmed. The fact is any invasive route is more likely to transmit this disease than dietary exposure. This includes sexual intercourse. It is well known that in the case of cattle that sperm can deliver the infection to an uninfected herd.

Scientific studies prove the connection. This is especially true of direct inoculation into the brain. Chimpanzees inoculated with diseased tissue from animals which die of mad cow-like diseases rapidly develop the disease, that is within a year or two. This raises the issue of the danger of vaccines grown on animal tissue as well as vaccines given to animals. The direct inoculation through contaminated vaccines may eventually be shown to play a greater role than feed or animal flesh in the spread of this disease. This is not to minimize the the significance of oral route as a factor: it is significant. Yet, direct inoculation is far more likely to rapidly precipitate the disease, in some cases within days or weeks of the insult. It was

Richard Rhodes, in his book *Deadly Feasts,* who claimed that the direct route, as occurs during surgery and vaccinations, increases the risks of contracting CJD a million-fold. This may explain the frighteningly high incidence of Alzheimer's disease, as well as Parkinson's disease and multiple sclerosis, in flu vaccine recipients.

The CJD agent remains largely unknown. Plus, it is persistent. It is well known that it may not be killed by routine sterilization. Thus, surgeries which expose brain or spinal cord tissue to the elements place patients at a heightened risk, especially if invasive devices are used. The greater the degree of invasion and the greater the number of instruments used, the higher the risk. Mere manipulation of the brain or severe head trauma also increases the risks: the agent, in fact, may exist in the normal brain. Severe brain trauma may dislodge it, precipitating the infection. The fact is the highest risk group for this disease is former brain surgery patients. Another high risk group is eye surgery patients due to the close proximity of this organ to the brain.

Meat is part of a healthy diet, that is healthy meat. Thus, there is nothing inherently wrong with it, that is if it is raised naturally. The fact is without it the body readily degenerates. There are certain substances in meat which cannot be procured through vegetation: for instance, vitamin B-12, vitamin D, and carnitine. Today, meat which is natural, as well as highly nourishing, is difficult to procure. Again, it is how the meat is raised, as well as prepared, that is the issue, not any inherent danger in it per se.

Numerous native tribes subsist primarily upon meat. Yet, such tribes thrive in robust health. The fact is as soon as such peoples adopt a modern diet they degenerate. So, it is far from the meat or animal products that is the issue. It is how such animals are raised–it is how animal products are prepared–that is responsible. Primitive peoples fare far worse on modern diets than their native meat, milk, cheese, yogurt, that is animal-food-rich diets. So, it is far from animal products that are the issue. Again, it is how the animals are fed, raised, butchered, processed, and handled: this is the source of the epidemic. The fact is brain degeneration secondary to food is exclusively a man-made disease. Human meddling has created this debacle. Native peoples, whose diets are mainly meat and animal products, fail to contract mad cow-like syndromes. In such people CJD, Alzheimer's disease, multiple sclerosis, and Parkinson's disease are essentially unknown. The fact is such syndromes are epidemic in Western countries, where animal raising practices are corrupt. Here, strict herbivores are fed as if carnivores, a diabolical practice. This unnatural animal rearing is the source of the epidemic, not the mere consumption of flesh. There is no Alzheimer's or CJD in native peoples, who eat only naturally raised meats.

If animals eat proper diets, their flesh is healthy. If they are fed noxious substances, their flesh will correspond, that is it will be noxious. Beef is inherently sterile, especially flesh cuts. True, it may be afflicted with parasitic infestations: there is always a risk for contracting parasites from raw meat. Yet, herbivores in their native state, that is when they eat their natural forage—vegetation—are, generally, free from infection. In other words, they fail to harbor any potentially serious diseases, which could harm humankind, the exception being parasites, which are killed by proper cooking.

Yet, in America the food supply is corrupted, and this is true of all components, including the meat and milk. This is largely due to farming practices. Modern feeding practices are atrocious. Herbivores are no longer herbivores. For decades in America animal parts have been fed to herbivores. These animal parts have been ground into feed with grain. In their greed for quick financial gain feed companies have gone to all extremes to create low cost products. Here, they have added every conceivable source of animal protein: road kill, dead fetuses, blood, internal organs, diseased animals, dead research animals, pets, and more. Recently, in France a major scandal was exposed. The French, who export duck meat throughout the world, were feeding these animals a most devious concoction: grain mixed with septic tank residue. That is septic tanks were scraped and the residue mixed with various feeds. For decades this was the "feed of choice" in fattening French ducks. Yet, there is no evidence that the practice has been completely curbed. Thus, people should avoid the consumption of duck breast, that is unless the source is obvious (and safe). In Switzerland an even more dire practice was uncovered: human cannibalism. People were unwittingly becoming cannibals through the consumption of animal flesh. At least two Swiss abortion clinics had for an unknown period disposed of human placentas in rendering plants, where they were converted to animal feed. The feed was then fed to pigs and chickens, perhaps dairy cows. Yet, on a far more significant scale tens of millions of humans, mostly in the Western world, have consumed beef, as well as pork and chicken, fed with animal parts as well as animal blood. Such a practice creates diseased meat, which is high in both foreign protein, that is prions, and bizarre germs. Then, humans eat this abnormal meat, increasing their risks for a variety of diseases. It may eventually be proven that Alzheimer's disease and Parkinson's disease are at least to some degree a consequence of the consumption of flesh-fed, that is contaminated, meat.

The contamination of the commercial animal supply may be far more rampant than is recognized. For instance, consider the Swiss, who failed to properly dispose of human remains and who, instead, "recycled" fetal tissue as animal feed. Switzerland was second to England in cases of mad cow disease in cattle herds. This is further proof of how, as a result of errant feeding practices, rather, unbridled greed, disaster can result. The Swiss turned their herds into cannibals, and, thus, caused social and financial disaster. Yet, greed overcame any justice: after promising to destroy hundreds of thousands of potentially infected cattle the Swiss government ground the remains and fed them to pigs and chickens. This further perpetuated the risk. The fact is it is far from merely beef and lamb that is at issue. Carlton Gadjusek, British researcher, claims that at least in Britain "...all the pigs are infected" as well as "...all the chickens fed on meat and bone meal." So, it is not merely beef that must be addressed. The individual must also know how other meats are raised before purchasing or eating. The fact is restrictions have been placed upon cattle feed, while few if any have been placed upon pig and chicken feed. Thus, beef is probably a safer choice than commercial pork or chicken.

Pork has other issues. Its intake increases the risks for a variety of diseases, including cancer, heart disease, and bizarre forms of arthritis, including rheumatoid arthritis. This may be largely due to the fact that pigs are a different type of animal biologically from, for instance, herbivores. Pigs are omnivores. Their diet is unpredictable. If a dead rat is found in the pen, they will eat it. They also eat feces. They consume all manner of soil creatures, including parasites and earthworms. They root in dirt and mud and as a result contract the germs found therein. Thus, the flesh of pigs is extensively contaminated, which may explain why, for instance, in the Qur'an flesh of pork is described as *rijis,* which means filthy. The prophets of antiquity prohibited the consumption of pork. The reason is to prevent human disease. Trichinosis is only one of many factors. The primary reason is the feeding practices of the animal, which are never purely vegetarian. Besides trichinosis there are hundreds of other infectious agents transmitted through the consumption of pork, including pork whipworm, which is similar to the germ found in the brains of CJD victims. What's more, pork flesh is exceptionally difficult to digest, while the flesh of cows and lambs, as well as poultry, is relatively easy to digest.

Pigs are far from immune to this disease. Transmission of neurological diseases from pigs is well established, for instance, the outbreak of meningitis in Malaysia. Here, some 110 people died of a violent type of meningitis, which was traced directly to the pigs raised there in intensive farms.

The brains of pigs, as well as pork livers, are readily infected with a wide range of germs. If these tissues are eaten, or rendered into animal feed for commercial cattle, human infection is likely. Pork consumption is linked to chronic disease, including chronic wasting or senility diseases. In 1985 a study reported in the American Journal of Epidemiology documented how the regular consumption of, for instance, ham, increased the risk of contracting prion-related diseases some 1000%. What's more, research indicates that heavy pork consumers suffer from an increased risk of both Parkinson's disease and Alzheimer's disease. Outbreaks of neurological disorders secondary to pork consumption are well established. However, such outbreaks, at least in the United States, have been largely covered up.

The establishment of prions as the true cause of mad cow has yet to be confirmed. This remains a theory. A more likely cause is sepsis, that is fulminant infection of the brain. The brain tissue itself confirms this. Consider the term "spongioform", which means in the form of a sponge. This means the brain has holes eaten into it. What else could do so, that is other than a pathogen: an active living germ, which feeds on brain tissue. The word encephalopathy means brain pathology, that is disease of the brain. Thus, germs are the most likely cause. The prions alone couldn't be the cause. Active brain infection must exist. This is highly plausible. Renderers utilize all conceivable sources for their goods: the guts of slaughtered animals,

animals dying from unknown causes, wild beasts, zoo animals, and animals killed by blunt trauma, including so-called road kill. Surely, such animals and/or animal parts are fully contaminated. What's more, animals of all types are rendered, even those of the carnivorous family, for instance, rodents, dogs, cats, and rats, which carry vast numbers of disease-causing pathogens.

Prions—disease-causing proteins from the nerve tissue of various animals—are vile. However, even more vile is sepsis, that is the contamination of the food supply due to unnatural, in fact, diabolical, feeding practices.

The purpose of such feeding practices is far from nutritional enhancement: it is purely for financial gain. As a result of the violation of the divine code dire consequences result. Due to such violations the human race is suffering an unlimited degree of agony. In the Qur'an the divine law remains intact. This should be evaluated regarding proper laws, that is regarding the rules for healthy dietary, eating, and hygienic habits. For instance, it prohibits the consumption of animals which die spontaneously, that is from causes unknown. Obviously, such animals are potentially diseased and, thus, their flesh is unhealthy. Anyone who consumes such flesh is vulnerable to contracting disease, which is largely infective. It also disallows the consumption of animals dying from blunt trauma. Such trauma fails to allow the blood to be dispersed. The blood pools in the organs, leading to microbial growth. Plus, blunt trauma may break the spinal cord and brain casings, allowing the seepage of prions and prion-like agents, as well as nerve tissue viruses, into the tissues. Carrion is also prohibited, that is animal carcasses, which are being fed upon by various carnivores. Yet, such carcasses may enter the food supply through a stealth means: animal feed, which is eaten by cattle, which, then, humans consume. Through this humans receive the dangerous pathogens of various carnivores, including crows, ravens, hawks, vultures, cats, dogs, skunks, rats, and wolves, which feed on the carcasses. What's more, the nerve tissue from the dead animals may end up in rendered products. If the flesh of animals that were fed such tissue is eaten prions from unrelated species will be ingested. This will wreak havoc in the brain, possibly leading to mad cow-like syndromes.

Regarding flesh it is the blood that is most toxic. For untold centuries people have been consuming internal organs. There is no known connection between such dietary habits and the disease. Today, the circumstances have changed. Toxicity, plus unnatural feeding practices, has rendered in most instances the internal organs unfit for human consumption, especially the brain and spinal cord. In the Western world, where cattle are fed animal parts and/or blood meal or where they were fed in such a manner in the past, it is nutritional suicide to eat brain/spinal tissue. Such tissue surely is contaminated with the mad cow-related pathogens, which would readily infect humans. This is what happened to the Asian cannibals, who ritually ate their human dead. Eating such flesh caused them to contract a fatal neurological disease. The same would be true of a human in the Western world who ate contaminated animal flesh. The source is irrelevant: it is the contamination that is the issue. What's more, it's the degree of contamination that is key, that is how many doses will the individual get.

Rendering is convenient for farmers, while having no benefit for the consumer. An animal dies. The farmer merely calls the rendering factory, which hauls the animal off. No one screens it to ensure it is free of contamination. Even if it has been contaminated, attacked by crows, hawks, or wild dogs, as long as it is a money-bearing carcass it is processed: no questions asked. The farmers get paid for the weight of the carcass and it is considered no further. This animal is then so-called rendered for use in hundreds of products, including foods. Soaps, make-up, creams, and animal feed all may be derived from it. Through this process dead and diseased animal tissue becomes the fodder for a host of animals, including house pets, cattle, pigs, chickens, turkeys, and horses. Yet, incredibly, many of the animals are strict herbivore. Of the aforementioned only pigs and chicken will eat flesh. A variety of products for human use are also derived, including, as mentioned previously, facial care products, detergent, hand creams, and soap. Animal feed is particularly at question. Both the rendered protein and fat, that is the tallow, which are derived from the carcasses of a wide range of animals, are also added to feed, including pet food. The latter is particularly contaminated, since, here, the lowest-level raw materials are used.

Yet, it is not merely the errant feeding practices which are responsible for diseased animals. It is also the vaccines. Animals are extensively vaccinated. What's more, such vaccines introduce a plethora of pathogens, which readily and permanently infect animal tissues. Such pathogens may be efficiently transferred into humans, that is through the consumption of contaminated meat. Vaccines for animals are big business. Billions of dollars are reaped by drug companies every year. Yet, there is no evidence that such vaccines make the meat safer for humans. Rather, the fact is vaccines can only add further sepsis. Thus, besides financial gain there is no reason for their persistent use.

Greed is destroying the human race. For mere material gain, as well as power, people are placing at risk the entire human race. Could there be a greater violation against the natural law—against common human decency—than that?

The feed industry has only one interest: profits. No regard is given to human health, that is the consequences of errant feeding practices. The fact is commercial feeding practices violate Nature. As a result only disaster looms. A massive epidemic is brewing and it is strictly due to the financial motives of the few. There are major profits in the sale of rendered animal parts. Little is paid for these wastes and, when the residues are sold in feed bags, the profits are high. The NRA's (National Renderers Association) Web site tells all: renderers reap up to $600.00 per hundred weight for a wide range of animal-derived matter, from porcine blood meal to beef connective tissue. Yet, many renderers include in such meal a certain percentage of renderings from other sources, including wild animals and even pets. Animals which are rendered by the mega-ton every day include cats, dogs, guinea pigs, skunks, opossums, raccoons, deer, zoo animals, and even snakes. All this is rendered, that is boiled down. The resulting proteins and fats are then formulated into feed: for use in pet and farm-animal foods.

Regarding beef and lamb these animals are strict herbivores. In nature they never eat meat. Left to their native diets their meat becomes inherently safe, in fact, nourishing. Forcing them to violate their own native ways, that is by force feeding animal-derived products, in effect, turning the animals into carnivores, results in disease. This is true both in the animals and those who eat them. Again, these unnatural feeding practices are applied merely for financial gain: there is no human benefit as a result of such feedings. The purpose is to increase the weight of the cattle in order to earn more per head. Certainly, the feeding of animal parts to herbivores fails to improve the nutritional quality or taste of the meat—there is no health benefit. Do not eat commercial meats of any type, which are raised on animal-derived feeds. What's more, the consumption of animals given vaccines should also be avoided. This is because the vaccines are animal-derived and, therefore, can contribute to the sepsis. If there is even a remote chance that a meat is fed flesh, do not eat it. One dose is sufficient to lead to a writhing, fatal disease. Only eat grass fed or organically raised meats. There is no evidence that such meat can transmit serious disease.

In the United States animal parts have been fed to other animals for decades, primarily pigs and chickens. In some instances cattle have also been fed such products, that is feed-lot cattle. Even today despite all the warnings some feed manufacturers skirt the law. This is because, while flesh has now been prohibited in cattle feed, blood is still allowed, as is bone meal, the latter being notoriously contaminated. Thus, blood/bone meal feeds are available, and, again, they are used primarily for pigs and chickens. Yet, certainly, some of this ends up in cattle, particularly dairy cows. In certain instances such feed may also be given to feed-lot cattle.

No one knows the precise cause of Creutzfeldt-Jakob syndrome, that is mad cow. What is known is that it is some factor or group of factors found within flesh as well as blood. More specifically, it is an agent found in brain and spinal cord tissue. In fact, this agent(s) attacks and destroys nerve cells throughout the brain and spinal cord. Yet, obviously, it is a kind of infectious agent, which in a stealth manner destroys nerve tissue.

As mentioned previously commercial meats are raised for profitability, never health. This is leading to dire consequences. The raising of meat, as well as slaughtering practices, should be carefully regulated to prevent the transmission of potentially fatal diseases. Public health should be the first consideration, not profits. Yet, slaughterhouses routinely violate the health codes in favor of profits. Meat which is diseased and/or unhealthy, even cancerous, routinely passes through the system. Plus, animals which suffer from infections may be difficult to screen. The infections remain in the meat and, thus, may be transmitted to humans. The blood residues, a true waste product, are never wasted. It is sold to feed companies, which, then, feed it to cattle, particularly pigs and chickens. A kind of blood based milk, made from cow blood, is fed to calves, particularly veal calves. Other residues unfit for human consumption are processed into pet food.

Divine law prohibits such dangerous practices. The Torah prescribes specific practices regarding butchering. In Islam there is an invaluable practice: the cutting of the throat of the animal to drain all blood. Obviously, such practices are meant to protect the human race from potential catastrophes such as the ones now facing Western countries. In Western practice animals are shot with a stun gun before the throat is cut. This is a dangerous practice, since such a gun splinters the skull and causes brain tissue to splatter into the bloodstream. This could lead to the spread of mad cow-like diseases into the flesh. Industry should consider the more traditional practice of slaughtering through the draining of the blood, since the latter largely harbors disease. This would greatly improve the health of the meat supply and reduce the risk for the transmission of mad cow-like syndromes.

It is a dire state of affairs that the food supply cannot be trusted. Yet, how could it be trusted? Little if anything is done exclusively for the people: all is done for profits. Corners are cut; processes skimped, and procedures skirted. The result is catastrophic. Mad cow is one such catastrophe.

Regarding CJD it is largely humankind which has perpetuated this disease. The majority of animals who get it are farmed. In other words, the disease is virtually nonexistent in naturally reared animals. Regarding wild animals, again, the majority of cases occur in ranch-raised animals. An entire disease, never before occurring in nature, mink spongioform encephalopathy, is the result of man-made interventions. This disease first occurred in ranch-bred mink. Researchers in the United States clearly proved the cause: not mere close quarters or the spread of natural disease but, rather, the feed. The fact is W. T. Hubbert in *Diseases Transmitted from Animals to Man* states categorically that it is the feed that is responsible: an entire epidemic, leading to unmerciful pain and devastation, all due to human blundering.

The same is true of mad cow, that is bovine spongioform encephalopathy. This is a bovine brain infection and/or disease, therefore, the term encephalopathy (*encephalo* meaning brain). This term implies "pathology of the cephalic or brain region". The pathology is largely due to infection. It is a kind of sepsis of the brain, the result of the consumption of septic meat. The meat becomes septic due to the feed: normally such meat is relatively sterile. Plus, the feed contains prions, which are neurologically-based proteins of a highly destructive nature. These prions are impossible to destroy with normal heating temperatures. These prions are directly absorbed into the blood, where they cause vast disturbances, ultimately leading to brain degeneration.

Prions are brain proteins—the *pr* in prion stands for protein, while the *in* represents infection, that is it implies that this protein is infectious. The fact is Richard Rhodes in his book, *Deadly Feasts*, describes how the normal brain contains these agents. Prions can arise from virtually any species: that is any species whose brains are rendered into cattle, hog, and chicken feed. Through such feeds farm animals become cannibals: of their own species' brain tissues, as well as the tissues of multiple other species, including perhaps pets and zoo animals.

Since the feeding practices are so widespread, virtually all commercial farm animals have become contaminated. This means that the majority of Westerners, particularly Americans, British, French, Swiss, and Canadians, may suffer from a degree of the infection. Yet, the feeding practices have yet to be curbed. The feed manufacturers have violated all codes of ethics, giving no consideration to the impact of their productions. With these manufacturers regardless of the process safety has never been the issue.

There is no moral standing in such businesses. All that matters is profits. Human risk is rarely if ever considered. If there is money to be made, it is produced and sold. Cover-ups are rife, and every attempt has been made to conceal the facts from the consumers. Incredibly, despite the proven dangers, even in the United States certain farmers feed their cattle, hogs, and poultry various rendered feeds, which contain the CJD-causing agents. True, since 1997 the FDA issued a ban against feeding animal parts to ruminants. Yet, some feed manufacturers and farmers have outright ignored it. Yet, it was no true ban: it was merely a labeling issue. Rendered animal protein was merely labeled: Do Not Feed to Ruminants. This failed to prohibit farmers from using it. Plus, despite this labeling there has been no enforcement. The fact is the factory-farming industry has turned commercial cattle into cannibals, feeding them materials rendered from their own species. This is a vile practice. As demonstrated by the human cannibal experience in Papau, New Guinea, the result must be brain infection. What's more, blood products, which are extensively contaminated with germs, are routinely fed to pigs and poultry, as well as calves, the latter being slaughtered for veal. Currently, calves are fed a fluid derived from blood, which is supposedly rendered from cattle. Such blood is hopelessly infested with germs. Plus, surely, such blood products contain the mad cow-inducing agent. Rendering simply means boiling. It is the boiling of animal material down to a paste. Yet, such an action fails to sterilize animal matter. This is because animals are contaminated with various types of microbes which are resistant to heat. These resistant forms are the spores as well as cysts. Their very purpose is to resist environmental destruction, and the majority of these are highly heat-resistant. There are billions of such spores in animal tissues. Consider hog flesh. It contains an enormous number of microbial spores and/or cysts. A few square inches of hog skin may contain tens of millions of such spores. The hide is one of the items which is rendered. Thus, the "indestructible" spores enter the rendering. The bacterial content alone on hog skin is unfathomable. According to Jensen's *Microbiology of Meat* a mere two square inches harbors up to 4,000,000,000 (four billion) bacteria. Many of these are spore-forming. Thus, they will not be destroyed through rendering.

There are other even more frightening concerns. This involves a kind of germ, in fact, found in the brains of CJD victims. This is the spirochete or corkscrew bacteria. Similar to the bacteria which causes syphilis the spirochete is found living within brain tissue and membranes. Normally, the brain is sterile. This means any organism found within it must be infective. It means that it is at least part of the cause, if not the primary cause, of the disease. Spirochetes are definitely an abnormal finding. F. Bastion, M.D., a prominent neuropathologist, has found such pathogens within the brain tissue of people who die of this disease. The source: rats and mice. In fact, this germ was originally found in mice, where it causes a fatal brain infection. Yet, how does such a germ enter in large numbers in the human brain—how could they be responsible for an entire epidemic? An earlier book, Ford's *Textbook of Bacteriology,* gives the answer. Spirochetes form spores, which are virtually indestructible. Certainly, they survive the rendering process. What else could there be besides cattle in the renderings? Dead rats and/or mice, perhaps? Certainly, there are also pig and chicken guts, which are fully contaminated, plus feces. In particular, pork guts are highly contaminated, containing billions of spirochetes every few inches. What about rat and mice droppings as well as urine? Yet, what of the remainders—waste, on cement floors—which is swept up or shoveled and then rendered? There would certainly be mice and rats occasionally within. Any mouse or rat in the vicinity would certainly feast on such residue, leaving behind urine and droppings, and, therefore, hopelessly contaminating these scraps. When such rendered protein, complete with the guts of a wide range of animals, including swine guts and feces, which are notoriously contaminated with germs and where untold trillions of such spirochetes reside, is fed to animals, especially herbivores such as sheep, goats, and cows, the spores are ingested. Warmed by the enormous and highly fertile ruminant gut they hatch and begin infecting the animal. Ultimately, they reach the brain, where they establish themselves by the billions, gradually consuming and destroying it, leading to the characteristic lesions that have a spongy appearance: holes, like Swiss cheese, like a natural sponge—the holes that only spirochetes, that is corkscrew bacteria, can make. There are those who claim that this spongioform brain damage is related to the immune system–a kind of internal self-destruction. Yet, the immune system is incapable of creating such holes. The holes must be created, that is by an active force. The brain cannot create them on its own. Since corkscrew pathogens are found there and since they are abnormal inhabitants, can there be any other conclusion other than this simple fact: they are caused by invasive bacteria capable of boring such holes.

Now, it is claimed, at least in the United States and Canada, rendered animal parts are never fed to cattle. However, it is fully admitted that an even more insidious practice is allowed: the feeding of animal blood and bone meal. The bone meal itself contains blood and tissue: the remnants of the bone marrow as well as any remaining flesh. The slaughtering process: wholesale contamination? Cattle are slaughtered using a stainless steel blade, which punctures the neck veins and arteries. The blade might originally have been sterile, yet it quickly becomes contaminated. Jensen has shown that the slaughtering process fully contaminates it. The blade used to slaughter the animals can never remain sterile. Once the throat is punctured, for a few seconds the blood still circulates, delivering any contaminates from the blade into the tissue, including the bone marrow. What's more, the marrow retains as much as 8% of the original blood. Thus, this blood is ground up as part of the meal. The blood itself, which collects after slaughtering, instead of being decontaminated, is reserved. This is then spray-dried and added to the bone meal. Then, it is fed to farm animals, primarily chickens and pigs. This may explain the findings of V. L. Wheeler, Ph.D., who discovered that the regular consumption of commercial chicken, particularly chicken livers, can result in dire consequences: infection of the human body by cancer-causing germs. The fact is according to Wheeler cancer victims are commonly chicken eaters. She made an analysis of chicken products. The livers were so extensively contaminated that she deemed them unfit for human consumption. She also found the cancer-causing germs in chicken flesh as well as commercial eggs. When she isolated these germs and inoculated them into test animals, they developed cancers.

This leads to an ominous conclusion. Anyone who regularly eats commercial meats is infected. This may explain why in countries where farmers only feed their cattle natural forage Alzheimer's disease, Parkinson's disease, and Creutzfeldt-Jakob disease, as well as multiple sclerosis, are exceedingly rare.

Regarding the potential spread of these diseases there needs to be zero tolerance. Whether through rendering or edible meat no sick animal should ever enter the public food supply. If an animal is diseased, its transmission to all who eat it is likely.

This is a basic fact of medicine. Over 100 years ago it was Koch who proved this. He injected the fluids from diseased animals into healthy ones. All the healthy animals developed the disease. Thus, anyone who has eaten contaminated meat or, particularly, has been injected with serums or vaccines derived from such animals, is at risk for developing the disease. This means that potentially millions of Westerners are infected. It means that the epidemic already exists and that virtually anyone could contract it.

Only a symptom analysis can bear evidence of this infestation. Take the following test to determine if you have the signs and symptoms of this dreaded disease. Add the points and tally your score.

Which of these symptoms applies to you?   points

1. aching of the legs 1
2. weakness of the legs 1
3. dizziness 2
4. numbness and/or tingling of the feet or hands 2
5. atrophy (wasting) of the leg muscles 3
6. atrophy (wasting) of the muscles
   of the hands/arms 3
7. loss of coordination 3
8. personality changes 2
9. difficulty or impossibility of keeping balance
   on one leg 3
10. clumsiness 1
11. difficulty with speech and/or slurred speech 3
12. memory loss, which is gradually worsening 3
13. bizarre behavior, including unexpected
    aggression 3
14. bizarre sensations on or in the body 2

15. distortion in the appearance of objects 3
16. hallucinations 3
17. delusional ideas (megalomania) 3
18. tremors 2
19. tightening or spasms of the muscles 2
20. rigidity of the body and/or body contortions 4
21. freezing of the joints 1
22. headaches 1
23. visual disturbances 1
24. sudden changes in vision or sudden loss in vision 2
25. numbness in the tips of the fingers 1
26. numbness in the bottom of the feet 1
27. exhaustion/tiredness 1
28. stamping of the feet 4
29. twisting and crimping of the toes 2
30. loss of bladder control (incontinence) 3
31. uncontrollable jerking of the body 5
32. blindness that occurs suddenly .2
33. impaired ability to make judgements 2
34. exceptionally difficult time falling asleep 1
35. sudden or gradual paralysis of a limb 3
36. startled, panicky appearance 2
37. unusually agitated or hostile behavior 2
38. stiffness and/or tightness of the spine 1
39. impaired judgement 1
40. impaired thinking 1
41. increasing loss of capacity to vocalize words 3
42. reflexes are exaggerated 2
43. hysterical behavior 2
45. confusion to the point of delirium 1
46. double vision 1
47. disorientation 1
48. twitching of facial muscles 1

49. sudden weight loss 1
50. confabulations, i. e. mindless babbling 2
51. dragging of a leg or foot (or foot drop) 3
52. drooling 1
53. can't hold head up or head tilts to one side
     (loss of the strength of the neck muscles) 2

Your Score _____

1 to 8 Points–Possible or Mild CJD (i. e. the human equivalent of mad cow): Your symptoms could be due to a variety of disorders and are not necessarily due to CJD. Yet, your score could indicate an early case of this syndrome. What's more, since degenerative diseases of the brain are one of the leading causes of death in the Western world there is no reason to take any chances. It could also indicate a host of other less serious chronic disorders. However, any degree of neurological symptoms is abnormal. Assume the worst. Treat the condition as if it is early CJD by taking the neurological purge. Take the Oreganol P73 Juice, one ounce daily. Take also the Oregacyn, one capsule twice daily along with the Neuroloft, two capsules twice daily.

9 to 16 Points–Probable or Moderate CJD: You are developing symptoms indicating brain infection by CJD or a CJD-like agent. Do not take any chances. Attempt to reverse all symptoms immediately.

Recent data indicates that one of the agents is a spiral-shaped, that is corkscrew, pathogen, known as a spirochete. This is the same type of pathogen which causes syphilis. It is critical that you purge your brain and spinal cord, as well as the rest of the internal organs, of any residues of such agents. The agents could be virus-like or they could be bizarre bacteria, such as spirochetes, which bore holes through brain tissue. There is also likely a parasitic component, for instance, human or animal amoebas, which readily infect the brain. Regardless of the agent such invaders must be destroyed before they cause further tissue damage. Left untreated the condition could worsen into full-blown mad cow-like syndrome. To treat this condition drink Oreganol P73 Juice, one or two ounces twice daily. Also, take the Oregacyn, two vega-caps twice daily, along with the Neuroloft formula, three capsules twice daily. The oil of oregano may also be applied, rubbed up and down the spine at night before bedtime.

17 to 29 Points–Severe CJD: Surely, you are suffering from brain infection and/or damage. The consequences could be dire, that is if no action is taken. Recent data proves that in CJD or CJD-like diseases definite bacteria are infecting the brain, including corkscrew bacteria similar to syphilis. It is critical to thoroughly purge all toxins and infectious agents from the brain, including corkscrew bacteria, viruses, amoebas, and abnormal prions. This can be achieved by an aggressive antiseptic purge. Drink the water soluble Oreganol P73 Juice, two or more ounces twice daily. Retain the juice in the mouth as long as possible before swallowing. Take the Oregacyn (original formula): three capsules two or more times daily. Also, take Neuroloft formula, four capsules two or more times daily. Using the SuperStrength oil of wild oregano rub up and down the spine once or more often daily, particularly before bedtime. Also, take the Rosemary Essence, at least two ounces twice daily. Avoid the intake of all substances which agitate the nervous system, including cocoa, chocolate, caffeine, coffee, iced tea, NutraSweet, food dyes, and MSG. However, do not go on a vegan diet permanently. This could lead to a sudden decline in health. Rather, eat a moderate amount of all categories of

food, relying on only organic and grass fed sources for meat and milk products. Consider also a liver purge to reduce the toxic load on the body; take LivaClenz, two or more capsules twice daily. As an additional purging agent take the GreensFlush, 20 or more drops twice daily.

30 to 43 Points–Extreme CJD: Follow the aforementioned advice. At this level of infestation brain damage is imminent, in fact, already occurring. To halt this process a massive effort must be made. What's more, the effort must be continuous. Plus, the appropriate diet must be followed and all toxins avoided. The consumption of all nerve-agitating food additives, particularly food dyes, MSG, and NutraSweet, must be strictly avoided. What's more, the intake of refined sugar must be curtailed. Drink the water-soluble Oreganol P73 Juice, two or more ounces twice daily. Ideally, drink a half bottle daily. Hold the juice in the mouth as long as possible before swallowing. Take the Oregacyn (original formula): two capsules two or more times daily. Also, take Neuroloft formula, four capsules twice daily. Using the SuperStrength oil of wild oregano rub up and down the spine once or twice daily before bedtime. Also, using a Q-Tip apply the oil to the inside of the inner nose (not the outside layer but up into the nose on the inside) Also, take the Essence of Rosemary, two or more ounces twice daily. Take also the Essence of Neroli Orange, which is highly beneficial for brain chemistry, two ounces twice daily in hot water, adding raw honey, if desired. This is a highly luscious aromatic drink, which acts directly upon the brain. Many illnesses with vague symptoms are misdiagnosed as various neurological and psychiatric disorders: the true cause, which is often microbial, is often missed. Thus, if there exist persistent symptoms, not due to mere stress or mental problems, CJD is a likely diagnosis. However, do not go on a permanent vegan diet. This

could lead to a sudden decline in health. A strict vegan diet, while providing a wide array of healthy vegetables and fruit, may itself lead to disease. Rather, eat a moderate amount of all categories of food. For meat and milk products rely exclusively on only organic and grass fed sources for meat and milk products. Consider also a liver purge to reduce the toxic load on the body; take LivaClenz, two or more capsules twice daily. As an additional purging agent take the GreensFlush, 20 or more drops twice daily.

44 points and above–Profoundly Extreme CJD: The diagnosis of the human variant of mad cow disease, that is Creutzfeldt-Jacob disease, is virtually assured. The fact is in the event of such a score the likelihood of brain infestation is extreme. The brain may be contaminated, in fact, infected, by a wide range of pathogens, including prion-related agents, stealth viruses, vaccine virus residues, bizarre forms of DNA, largely from genetically engineered foods and vaccines, spirochetes, amoebas, sexually transmitted germs, and uncountable others. For health to be revived all must be purged from the brain and spinal cord as well as the remaining tissues. A multiple-pronged therapy is required. Take the Oreganol P73 Juice, as much as possible daily: even a bottle daily. Take also Oregacyn, four capsules with food or heavy juice three or four times daily. Also, take the Neuroloft-Mind formula, four capsules three times daily. As an additional healing agent, that is for regenerating damaged nerve endings, take the crude red grape powder, that is the Resvital, one heaping teaspoon twice daily or as capsules, four twice daily. Also, drink the Rosemary Essence, three ounces twice daily. To strengthen the glands, which are weakened by such a systematic disease, take the Royal Power, four capsules twice daily. Also, using a Q-Tip apply the Oreganol oil of wild oreganol to the inside of the inner nose (not the outside layer but

up into the nose on the inside). The CJD agent has been found residing on the inside of the nose. Therefore, it also resides in the sinuses. This may be purged out of this region through the Q-Tip approach along with taking the oil under the tongue twice or more daily. However, do not go on a permanent vegan diet. This could lead to a sudden decline in health. Rather, eat a moderate amount of all categories of food, relying on only organic and grass fed sources for meat and milk products. Consider also a liver purge to reduce the toxic load on the body; take LivaClenz, two or more capsules twice daily. As an additional toxic chemical and liver purge take the GreensFlush, 40 or more drops twice daily.

Evaluating the risks: the Risk Assessment Questionnaire

There is another means to assess the status. This is the Risk Assessment Questionnaire. This tells if the individual is already inoculated with the CJD agents. In other words, it is a sign of significant risk for the future development of this disease. In the United States the potential of undiagnosed or early CJD is high. Errant animal feeding practices have created an endemic infection, plus surgical procedures, as well as vaccines, have introduced such agents into the population. Thus, a means to determine early manifestations of this disease or, in fact, the existence of hidden infections, will prove invaluable.

This is an epidemic of proportions beyond comprehension. There are some one million deaths from CJD globally, primarily in the Western world. Estimates vary but in the United States alone there may be as many 250,000, perhaps 500,000, active cases. Others have estimated the CJD or CJD-like cases to be as high as 2,000,000. This is far from an overestimate. With the increasing administration of genetically engineered vaccines, which harbor animal-source pathogens, the risks for developing CJD are exceedingly high. This means that in the United States every year potentially thousands of individuals are likely dying from syndromes similar to mad cow. The majority are given a vague diagnosis—Alzheimer's, Parkinson's, encephalitis, or multiple sclerosis—and the true cause is never determined. However, merely avoiding commercial meat products is only part of the answer. There are even more noxious sources of these germs: invasive therapies, particularly spinal and brain surgery as well as vaccines. Invasive dentistry is another significant source. Early research in the 1950s demonstrated how the dentist's drill could rapidly precipitate brain infections, which could, ultimately, lead to chronic disease. These are the most likely sources for fulminant mad cow-like syndromes in humans.

RISK ASSESSMENT TEST

The following is a means of assessing the risks for developing CJD, that is the human form of mad cow disease. Again, since there is no definite blood or medical test historical analysis is required. The results of this questionnaire may demonstrate an ominous finding: the existence of incubating CJD, that is the disease is being harbored and may break out: at any moment. Add up the score for your total.

Which of these apply to you?   **points**

1. To what degree have you had invasive
   dentistry during your lifetime?
   a) one to two events 2
   b) three to four events 3

c) five to seven events 5
d) eight or more events 7

2. Have you had root canals?
a) one. 2
b) two to three 3
c) four to five 4
d) six or more 6

3. Do you consume aspartame on a daily
   or weekly basis? 1

4. Do you consume large quantities of aspartame
   such as several diet sodas daily? 2

5. Have you had invasive brain surgery? 5

6. Have you had spinal taps? 1

7. Have you had bone marrow taps? 2

8. Have you undergone bone marrow transplants? 3

9. Have you had a corneal transplant? 2
10. Have you undergone cataract surgery? 2

11. Do you eat raw beef or pork from commercial
    sources on a regular basis? 3

12. Do you eat commercial or feed-lot beef
    on a regular basis? 2

13. Do you eat commercial chicken or pork
    on a regular basis? 2

14. Do you eat brain or spinal cord tissue,
    or have you eaten it in the past? 3

15. Do you drink alcoholic beverages on a regular basis? . . .3

16. Were you formerly a heavy drinker? 2

17. Do you regularly eat hot dogs? .2

18. Are you taking potent mind-altering drugs
on a regular basis? 2
(add 3 additional points if taking two or more such drugs)

19. Are you under the care of a psychiatrist
for a severe mental illness? 1

20. Have you been hospitalized for a mental illness? 1

21. Do you have a family history of Alzheimer's
or Parkinson's disease? 3

22. Do you currently have Alzheimer's
or Parkinson's disease? 5

23. Has anyone in your family had CJD
or similar destructive neurological diseases? 5

24. Do you have multiple sclerosis? .3

25. Have you received blood transfusions?
a) one transfusion 2
b) two to three transfusions 3
c) four to six transfusions 4
d) seven or more transfusions 7

26. Have you had the flu vaccine?
a) once 4
b) two to three times 6
c) four to five times 8
d) six to seven times 10
e) eight or more 12

27. Have you had all the traditional vaccines
of childhood? 5

28. Have you had the hepatitis and/or
meningitis vaccines? 5

29. Are you a heavy consumer of commercial beef? 4

30. Do you eat large amounts of commercial chicken? 2

31. Are you a frequent pork eater? 3
31. Do you eat commercial lamb or lamb chops often? 3

Your Score _____

---

1 to 4 points–Possible inoculation: There is a remote possibility that you are inoculated with the CJD agents. As a preventive measure avoid the intake of commercial meats. Instead, consume farm-fresh naturally raised meats such as grass-fed beef and lamb as well as free-range poultry. As a preventive tonic take Oregacyn, one capsule daily.

5 to 11 points–Probable inoculation: the probability is significant that you have been inoculated with the CJD agents. A purge is required. Take the Oreganol P73 Juice, one or two ounces daily. Take also Oregacyn, one or two capsules twice daily. Take the Neuroloft formula, 2 capsules daily. Avoid all commercial meats. Instead, consume farm-fresh naturally raised meats such as grass-fed beef and lamb as well as free-range poultry.

12 to 19 points–Mild-Moderate inoculation: You are at a significant risk for the development of dementia syndromes, including the mad cow variant, CJD, as well as multiple sclerosis. Avoid the intake of commercial meats and eat instead naturally raised meats, which are never fed animal protein. Follow the advice for the purge in the moderate CJD section. What's more, take LivaClenz, as well as the GreensFlush, to purge toxins from the liver and ease the body's toxic burden.

20 to 27 points–Severe inoculation: Infestation by the CJD agents is virtually assured. Follow the aforementioned advice.

Untreated, a fulminant neurological disease could develop. This may be manifested by chronic symptoms, which might cause the individual to seek psychiatric care. Thus, depression, mania, psychosis, and anxiety may be, in fact, undiagnosed or early CJD. The risk is also exceedingly high for the development of multiple sclerosis and myasthenia gravis. The so-called muscular dystrophy epidemic may also be vaccine-induced, since the vaccine toxins can be transported to the fetus through the sperm and egg. Eliminate the risk for developing this disease by consuming high doses of potent spice extracts. Follow the advice in the former section under extreme CJD infection. Be sure to avoid all commercial beef, chicken, and pork and, instead, consume naturally raised meat. Grass-fed beef and lamb are ideal. Massive doses of purging agents are necessary. Take the Oreganol P73 Juice, two ounces twice daily. Hold this in the mouth as long as possible before swallowing. Also, take the Oregacyn, two capsules three times daily with meals. The oil must also be taken, about 10 drops under the tongue twice daily. The Neuroloft is a powerful aid: take three capsules twice daily. What's more, take LivaClenz, as well as the GreensFlush, to purge toxins from the liver and ease the body's toxic burden.

28 to 33 points–Extreme inoculation: Infestation by the CJD agents, that is the agents which cause destructive damage to the brain, is virtually assured. Thus, the risk for developing CJD or various dementia syndromes, such as Alzheimer's and/or Parkinson's, is exceptionally high. The risk is also exceedingly high for the development of multiple sclerosis and myasthenia gravis. The so-called muscular dystrophy epidemic may also be vaccine-induced, since the vaccine toxins can be

transported to the fetus through the sperm and egg. Eliminate the risk for developing this disease by consuming high doses of potent spice extracts. Follow the advice in the former section under extreme CJD infection. Be sure to avoid all commercial beef, chicken, and pork and instead consume naturally raised meat. Grass-fed beef and lamb are ideal. Massive doses of purging agents are necessary. Take the Oreganol P73 Juice, two to four ounces twice daily. Hold this juice in the mouth as long as possible before swallowing. Also, take the Oregacyn, two capsules three times daily with meals. The oil must also be taken, about 10 drops under the tongue twice daily. The Neuroloft is a powerful aid: take three capsules twice daily. What's more, take LivaClenz, as well as the GreensFlush, to purge toxins from the liver and ease the body's toxic burden.

34 to 43 points–Exceptionally extreme inoculation: You have a vast degree of risk for inoculation with the CJD agent(s). Most likely, this agent(s) already exists in your tissues. The agent could cause a wide range of neurological disorders, including Alzheimer's disease, dementia, Parkinson's disease, and multiple sclerosis. All could be, in fact, CJD, which was mis-diagnosed. Aggressively purge such agents from your tissues and from your nervous system. With this degree of invasive exposure, certainly, your tissues are under the burden of multiple infections by a wide range of pathogens, many of which are attacking the brain and spinal cord. Massive doses of purging agents are necessary. Take the Oreganol P73 Juice, two or more ounces twice daily. Hold this juice in the mouth as long as possible before swallowing. Also, take the Oregacyn, three capsules three times daily with meals. The oil must also be taken, about 20 drops under the tongue two or three times daily. The Neuroloft is a powerful aid: take three capsules three times

daily. Be sure to avoid all commercial beef, chicken, and pork and instead consume naturally raised meat. Grass-fed beef and lamb are ideal. Halt the consumption of all commercially raised meat and fowl. The Essence of Rosemary, as well as the Essence of Neroli Orange, is invaluable. Take an ounce twice daily of each. Also, take the crude red grape powder, that is the Resvital, a heaping teaspoon twice daily. What's more, take LivaClenz, as well as the GreensFlush, to purge toxins from the liver and ease the body's toxic burden.

44 points and above–Profoundly extreme inoculation: Surely, your brain and spinal tissues have been inoculated with the CJD agent(s). Most likely, this agent(s) is actively infecting your tissues, causing a massive degree of brain damage. The agent could cause a wide range of neurological disorders, including Alzheimer's disease, dementia, Parkinson's disease, and multiple sclerosis. You may already suffer from such a disease. All could be, in fact, CJD, which was misdiagnosed. Aggressively purge such agents from your tissues and from your nervous system. With this degree of invasive exposure, certainly, your tissues are under the burden of multiple infections by a wide range of pathogens, many of which are attacking the brain and spinal cord. Massive doses of agents capable of purging the nerve tissues are necessary. Take the Oreganol P73 Juice, three or more ounces twice daily. Hold this juice in the mouth as long as possible before swallowing. Also, take the Oregacyn, three or more capsules three times daily with meals. The oil must also be taken, about 20 drops under the tongue three or more times daily. The Neuroloft is a powerful aid: take four capsules three times daily. Be sure to avoid all commercial beef, chicken, and pork and instead consume naturally raised meat. Grass-fed beef and lamb are ideal. Halt the consumption of all commercially raised meat

and fowl. The Essence of Rosemary, as well as the Essence of Neroli Orange, is invaluable. Take two ounces twice daily of each. Also, take the crude red grape powder, that is the Resvital, a heaping teaspoon twice daily. What's more, take LivaClenz, as well as the GreensFlush, to purge toxins from the liver and ease the body's toxic burden.

Preventive advice

Treatment of this condition should initially be preventive. Every effort should be made to avoid the intake of commercial meats, opting instead for meats raised with known growing practices. Kosher and Islamic meats are also available. Grass-fed and organic meats are additional options. The point is all such options are superior to commercial meats.

Tell your grocer that you will no longer buy beef or lamb, that is unless you know the source: unless it is organic or grass-fed. Grain-fed animals might appear to be another option. They are not. This is because the grains are largely genetically engineered, and this process also introduces animal contaminants as well as toxic germs. Avoid all beef, lamb, or poultry which is fed such grains. Tell your grocer that unless he/she can guarantee that the animals are fed naturally—without animal parts, bone meal, blood meal, or genetically engineered grains, you will not buy it. Get their attention. This will help not only yourself but also ensure the future for your children and loved ones. The quality of the food supply in America must change. Otherwise, the consequences will be catastrophic: the end of civilization as we know it.

The pathogen(s) should also be destroyed. This requires aggressive therapy. The key is to get enough medicine to cross the blood-brain barrier. Follow the advice in the CJD questionnaire. The key components are Oregacyn, the Juice, and the oil as well as the Neuroloft. In general take as much of these items as necessary to achieve results. These are safe spice extracts and enormous doses are safe. The CJD agents are difficult to reverse and this is why mega-dosing is critical. Also, take a potent wild greens supplement, that is the GreensFlush, two droppersful under the tongue twice daily. (Note: The GreensFlush drops can only be ordered via mail order: 1-800-243-5242 or in Canada, 866-776-6550.) Also, in tough cases perform spice oil rubs. Using Oreganol SuperStrength, along with, perhaps, edible oil of clove buds and/or sage, rub the entire back and spine twice daily. Also, rub the SuperStrength up and down the lower and upper legs over the long bones. Using a Q-Tip saturated with the oil place this up along the inside of the nasal membranes (not the more sensitive outer membranes; allow to contact the membrane as long as possible). Do this daily to get the oil directly into the sinuses, where the CJD agent frequently resides. Other substances which may be of value include Essence of Rosemary, Essence of Rose Petals, Essence of Neroli Orange, and Wild Oregano Honey.

There can be no harm from aggressive natural therapy. The fact is there is harm from the disease, that is if there is no stopping the progression, the individual will die. Thus, a major effort with the oil, juice, Oregacyn, GreensFlush, etc. is crucial. The fact is it will likely prove lifesaving.

It is a true debacle to have to correct, that is resolve, human misery. It is much more constructive to prevent such catastrophes. It is mere greed and lust for more that causes people to overstep the boundaries, that is the limits of common decency. Humanity must reduce its aggression, which only leads to self destruction. There must be a change. Otherwise, all will be lost and humanity itself may suffer extinction.

The quality of the food supply in America must be improved. The general public can assist this process through their buying power. People must show force immediately to attempt to reverse the tyranny, that is the arrogance of forcibly changing nature. The fact is scientists are forcibly altering a code, which is highly sophisticated and which could never otherwise be altered.

The genetic code of each animal is sanctified; the animal natively resists any possibility of genetic corruption. Consider the lowly colonic bacteria, E. coli. For decades scientists have attempted to manipulate this bacteria to accept foreign genetic material: it refused. Only through forcibly altering the bacteria's structure—by shocking it with chemicals, electricity, and extremes of heat and cold—only then did the bacteria take up the foreigners. In other words, only after the germ was weakened and corrupted—that was the beginning of genetic engineering. This is no science. It is pure raw corruption. Now, the engineered food is forced upon the people. Virtually no one in the United States accepts such food as legitimate. No one wishes to knowingly eat it. Yet, this corrupt food has penetrated all realms of the food supply. It is disease producing. It should be avoided at all costs.

The people must fight for their rights and resist all forms of tyranny. Otherwise, the consequences will be catastrophic: the end of civilization as we know it.

Yet, it is important to realize that there is no reason to give up hope. According to the premise of this book CJD is a septic contamination of the brain. Thus, if the sepsis is neutralized, that is if the pathogens are destroyed, the tissue can heal. In the late 1800s arsenic-based compounds were used to destroy brain infections. Today, spice extracts, which are safe, offer this power. If the brain infection is halted, the body may be able to eliminate the abnormal prions. What's more, once the brain infection is halted, the bizarre and frightening symptoms will dissipate. The key is penetration, that is of the medicine to cross the blood-brain barrier. This is achieved through the powers of multiple spice extracts. However, the most essential items are the essences, that is the Oreganol P73 Juice. This tonic directly crosses the blood-brain barrier, offering a direct action against the CJD agent. Thus, it is the premier substance for neutralizing this disease. Be sure to take the Oreganol P73 Juice regularly at least three times daily. Also, hold it in the mouth as long as possible before swallowing. This may also be used as a nasal wash, or it may simply be inhaled through the nose. The regular use of Oreganol P73 Juice offers the capacity to reverse, as well as prevent, this disease. There is no harm in it. It can even be given to babies and pets.

Mold

This is certainly a global dilemma. In the United States it is a dire epidemic. Mold has contaminated innumerable buildings and homes, causing health problems for millions of people. Here, unseasonably warm weather patterns have accelerated the growth of molds, both outdoors and indoors. Plus, floods have damaged homes and other buildings, leading to mold contamination. In some instances vast amounts of mold have grown in hidden regions, that is under carpets or inside of walls or ceilings, causing extreme health problems in the inhabitants.

Mold is highly toxic. It can cause virtually any type of symptom or disease.

While it is little known mold plays a significant role in the development of global epidemics. It is an insidious factor. For instance, in many parts of the United States there has been an inordinate amount of rain, which breeds molds. Once within the body these molds suppress immunity. This is largely because molds produce a number of chemicals, which are among the most potent immunosuppressive compounds known.

The weather is highly abnormal. The poles are melting. Weather patterns, previously predictable, are changing dramatically. It seems that nothing is predictable. There is also a lack of truly cold weather, that is a normal winter which is needed to destroy airborne and soil molds. The lack of truly cold weather allows the molds to breed unchecked. The result is abnormally high mold levels and contamination of the air, soil, vegetation, buildings, homes, and, ultimately, humans as well as pets and other animals.

The lack of freezing weather in areas which are normally frigid is a serious dilemma. As a result, molds grow voluminously, invading a wide range of man-made and natural structures. The mold count in the air remains inordinately high, especially in areas where there is significant moisture.

There has been an epidemic of mold infections in children. This is apparently largely due to the contamination of school buildings by molds. Thus, children enduring such contamination are prime candidates for SARS and/or pandemic flu. The fact is children who die suddenly in school could be victims of toxic mold exposure. Mycotoxins are potent poisons. A rather insignificant amount can be sufficiently potent to cause sickness, even death. In fact, any child who dies suddenly from an unknown cause must be evaluated as a potential mold victim.

Few people realize it but the bubonic plague was associated with mold. According to Matossian in her book *Poisons of the Past: Mold Epidemics and History* wet weather during that era in Europe led to mold contamination of the grain. Both people and animals consumed this grain. This greatly weakened their immune systems, making them highly vulnerable to the plague bacteria. It also increased their vulnerability to viral and fungal infections. This same debacle occurred to the people of Pharaoh, when their grain was contaminated by flooding. Yet, this is precisely the circumstance in much of America: there is extensive flooding and the weather is unseasonably warm. Thus, in North America mold infestation is epidemic.

In suppressing the immune system mold toxins are so potent that if the intoxication is widespread, a pandemic is a virtual certainty. This is precisely the scenario in America today. It's not just one cause alone that could account for a global killer. There must be numerous factors. In fact, there will likely be several outbreaks, virtually simultaneously. Thus, it is usually a combination of events, even a combination of germs and/or toxins, which accounts for such a high degree of compromise. Everyone is searching for the single cause, the one culprit. It's rarely that simple. If it were not for the disruption of the ecosystem, as well as generalized toxicity to human health, such as can occur from mass vaccination, as occurred during the early 20th century, that is as a result of WW I, then such massive global killers would likely never arise.

The germ(s) are given too much credit, in fact, too much power. They are far from all-powerful. The fact is germs are rather weak. They are conquerable, that is if you understand what you are dealing with and know how to treat it. Yet, it is easy to understand why they are so extensively feared. Medicine offers no hope for a cure. Medical experts often create a sensation of hopelessness, in fact, fear. Too much power is given to the disease agent, largely because physicians themselves feel a kind of negativity, even despair. Thus, between the fear-mongering of the media and the hopelessness of the medical profession, no wonder people are frightened. Yet, then, if a person failed to understand the cause and, what's more, knew of no cures there would only be fear.

Molds produce a highly potent group of substances known as mycotoxins. The amount of such toxins on the tip of a pin is enough to kill an individual. Mycotoxins disrupt the function of the internal organs. They are particularly toxic to nerve tissue, including the brain. The fact is the intake of such toxins has been associated with a variety of brain diseases, including senility disorders, multiple sclerosis, manic-depressive syndrome, schizophrenia, and Parkinson's disease. There may even be an association between mycotoxins and mad cow disease or its human equivalent, Cruetzfeldt-Jakob (CJD) disease. Regarding CJD, that is the human form of mad cow disease, there are a number of causes. Obviously, contaminated grain, when consumed, will contaminate the cattle. While prions have been implicated as the cause of human mad cow disease molds could well be a "hidden" factor. This is because these germs produce potent toxins, which directly damage brain tissue. Plus, such toxins weaken the immune system, increasing the risks for the development of CJD-like diseases. It is certainly true of Alzheimer's. What's more, the latter is a variant of CJD. The diseases are, in fact, very similar.

If grain is contaminated with mold, so is the cattle, which consumes it. Mycotoxins are concentrated in the organs and flesh. A person who eats the contaminated meat also becomes contaminated. The mycotoxins are potent neurotoxins. Could this be the connection between animal product consumption, grains, and mad cow disease? Only further investigation will tell. Certainly, however, there is a connection. This is because the removal, particularly, of commercial grain, as well as grain-fed cattle products, from the diet of patients with senility diseases frequently leads to an improvement in this disease.

Mold is a pervasive germ. It is a major cause of sickness and even death. It vigorously invades human surroundings, since it readily grows on organic and even inorganic surfaces. Moisture, darkness, coolness, and food are its vital requirements. It can grow on virtually any food. It is found in the majority of homes, especially those with crawl spaces, basements, or attics. Any home which is dark or damp is mold-contaminated.

Obviously, there is a need for a substance which safely kills mold. Natural mold killers, which are non-toxic on common surfaces, would prove invaluable. The need is also for a safe substance which consistently reduces mold counts, perhaps eliminates them. Such a substance must also be safe for children and pets. Germ-a-Clenz is a potent natural germicide, which readily kills molds, both in the air and as well as on surfaces. Plus, it is edible, which means it can be used to reduce mold counts on or in the body. Thus, it is safe to use, even near babies and pets. Essentially, Germ-a-Clenz is a water-soluble form of wild oregano oil plus other antifungal spice oils, including edible oils of cumin and cinnamon.

Many people are familiar with the mold-killing powers of oil of wild oregano. The fact is it is a potent mold killer. Research by Akgul and Kivanc showed that the oil not only kills all molds but also destroys mold toxins. Beroud found that it inactivated aflatoxin, the most potent mold poison known. At Georgetown University oil of wild oregano (P73 Oreganol) was found to specifically destroy Candida albicans, a major cause of human disease. This yeast was destroyed both in the test tube and living tissue. A study by the FDA found that oil of wild oregano kills food-borne molds, that is the molds which spoil food. At a private lab researchers discovered that an aerosolized type of wild oregano oil, that is the Germ-a-Clenz, killed airborne molds as well as their spores. The latter study indicates that such an aerosol would be infinitely valuable for people allergic to airborne molds, especially asthmatics. Germ-a-Clenz itself fails to elicit allergic reactions, rather, it eliminates them by cleansing the air. In fact, inhaling the mist tends to open up clogged sinuses. Mold or fungal infection is another significant risk factor. Molds and various fungi, including yeasts, readily infect the body. There is an epidemic of infections by these organisms. As mentioned previously global warming and an increase in flooding are major contributors to the increased exposure to mold. Of the various types of fungi molds are perhaps the most insidious. There is a virtual pandemic of mold infections in many regions of North America. Molds usually enter the body through inhalation, although both molds and mold toxins may also be ingested. Ultimately, the molds enter the body, that is the blood and/or organs, where they multiply, causing infection and, ultimately, disease. The mycotoxins in particular may also enter the brain, where they disrupt brain chemistry, increasing the risks for central nervous system diseases. This is why in many instances people with neurological diseases improve dramatically if grains, which are typically contaminated with mycotoxins, are removed from the diet.

A vast number of molds are now known to infect the body. They may invade virtually any organ and readily infect both the digestive tract and bloodstream. These molds include aspergillus, penicillium, stachybotrus, cladosporidium, and fusarium. Microbiologists have found various molds in the bloodstreams of relatively normal people. However, the counts of these molds are highest in people who are chronically ill. Diseases associated with mold infection of the blood include chronic fatigue syndrome, polymyositis, fibromyalgia, arthritis, lupus, migraine headaches, ankylosing spondylitis, schizophrenia, bronchitis, asthma, and chronic sinusitis. CJD has yet to be associated, but in many cases a careful history with such patients will determine a connection. However, a thorough study must be done to determine the potential role of mold infection in the genesis of this disease. Yet, in Alzheimer's disease there is a connection: the ingestion of corn and other mycotoxin-contaminated foods. Thousands of Alzheimer's victims have a history of massive corn consumption. The fact is commercial corn is the primary food which is mold contaminated. Another heavily contaminated food, peanuts, is also a frequent item on Alzheimer's patient's menus.

The fact is a large percentage of individuals who develop this disease are addicted to peanuts and/or peanut butter. Yet, the role of allergy to corn and/or to mycotoxin-contaminated corn is even more significant, as is demonstrated by the following:

Case History:

Mr. H. was a 54-year-old male with a history of early Alzheimer's disease. He had lost the ability to drive and couldn't read a map. His ability to think clearly was also lost: he had no short-term memory. His wife had to perform most of his personal tasks, including dressing and feeding him, as well as driving him, for instance, to the clinic. She asked for his help in reading the map but he was incapable. On taking a history I determined he was addicted to breakfast cereals, mostly corn-based, as well as canned corn, corn chips, and similar grain-based foods. His diet was dramatically changed: no corn and, in fact, no grains, were allowed. He improved dramatically, primarily because of eliminated corn- and sugar- based foods. By his next visit, a mere three weeks, he was able to drive on his own: without his wife or a map.

Molds, as well as mycotoxins, enter the body through a variety of means: through the food, air, water, and skin. Once these molds become established in the body they greatly depress the immune system. Mycotoxins, which are highly toxic, even in miniscule amounts, especially against the immune cells but also against the endocrine cells. These substances readily disrupt cell chemistry, weakening the resistance against disease. In only minute quantities they may cause significant immune suppression. The fact is mycotoxins are among the most potent immunosuppressive substances known. Matossian, in her book, *Poisons of the Past: Mold Epidemics and History*, correlates exposure to such toxins as a primary cause of catastrophic plagues. The various major pandemics of history, which have led to the decline and/or collapse of civilizations, are apparently due in part to mold and, therefore, mycotoxin, poisoning. The molds and mycotoxins poisoned the people, largely as a result of the ingestion of wet/contaminated grain, leading to a generalized depression of the immune system. In other words, the mycotoxins poisoned the ability of the white blood cells to destroy germs. The toxins had a generalized depressive effect upon the immune system. The immune systems of such weakened individuals became so vulnerable that massive plagues readily developed.

Mycotoxins essentially neutralize the immune system. They also disrupt the hormone system and are particularly toxic to the reproductive system. This was demonstrated by a recent poisoning in animals. Both cows and pigs in Iowa are becoming infertile from eating corn. The corn is genetically engineered. This engineering weakens the corn's immune system, making it highly vulnerable to mold infection. The engineered corn, which was fed to the animals, was found to be infected with fusarium fungus. Apparently, the mycotoxins from this fungus had fully contaminated the corn. When the corn was eaten, it completely disrupted the reproductive systems of the pigs and cows, rendering them infertile. Interestingly, when one of the farmers reverted to feeding the cattle non-genetically engineered corn, the reproductive problems disappeared. Thus, not only were the fungal toxins causing the sickness but, apparently, some unknown contaminant in the genetically engineered corn is also poisoning these animals.

Corn, whether organic, genetically engineered, or 'regular', is notoriously contaminated with mold. This is largely a result of farming practices. If the corn is stored in silos, mold may readily grow. If it is air dried and then properly packaged, mold will not grow. For mold to grow moisture plus darkness is required. Plus, mold readily grows on sugar. Thus, any food which is relatively high in it will support mold growth. Of all vegetables corn is highest in sugar. Fruit also readily grows mold, the high sugar fruits being most vulnerable. Fruit highest in sugar includes grapes, apples, pears, raisins, dates, figs (dried), and pears. Low sugar fruit includes grapefruit, lemons, limes, strawberries, papaya, kiwi, and melons.

Yet, there is another factor: rat and mouse droppings. There is extensive contamination of commercial grain, corn, soybeans, and wheat with such droppings, as well as urine. Such wastes certainly contain germs, which may also account for the severe allergies and intolerance people exhibit against such foods.

There are a number of ways an individual can be exposed to mold. These exposures include mold growth on food, in refrigerators, in homes, in gutters (when cleaning them), in basements, in office buildings, in old books, and uncountable others. What's more, certain drugs increase the growth of molds, notably antibiotics and cortisone. So does sugar. A mere teaspoon or so daily dramatically increases mold counts in the blood. This indicates the commonness of mold infections. Signs and symptoms of mold infection include runny nose, post nasal drip, sinus pressure, stuffy sinus, sinus headache or pain behind the eye, achy head, nose bleeds, joint aches, wheezing, chest congestion, ticklish cough, exhaustion, depression, muscle aches, and hives.

Mold may readily grow on virtually any food, that is except meat, eggs, and milk. For instance, nuts and seeds may contain high mold levels. Certain foods are relatively resistant to mold growth, for instance, hot spices such as mustard, cumin, sage, cayenne, garlic, oregano, bay leaf, and thyme. Yet, incredibly, both onions and garlic may sustain mold growth. Besides corn various grains are major sources of mold. The grains which are most vulnerable include wheat and rye. For those who are mold sensitive avoidance of corn, wheat, and rye is critical. To neutralize mycotoxins raw nuts and seeds may be gently roasted for a few minutes on low heat (i.e. 150 to 200 degrees). Wild or brown rice may be eaten as a starch source instead of commercial grains. To reduce exposure to mold eat only low sugar fruit such as grapefruit, kiwi (hard), watermelon, cassava, lemons, limes, blueberries, and fresh strawberries.

Mold contamination can be reduced through the use of spice extracts. Germ-a-Clenz multiple spice extract spray is ideal for this purpose. Simply spray on the outside of any suspect fruit and wipe. Or, spray directly into fruit and simply leave. The latter approach is ideal for strawberries, raspberries, blueberries, currants, blackberries, raisins, figs, dates, and similar soft or watery fruit. It may also be used to decontaminate fruit with hard outer surfaces. For instance, cantaloupe is an ideal fruit for the mold sensitive person, since it is low in sugar. However, it tends to develop mold infections on the surface. This is where Germ-a-Clenz is ideal. Simply spray on the cantaloupe and allow to sit. Rinse or leave to dry. Then, after an hour or two cut and serve. Watermelon may also be contaminated, because of its direct connection with the ground. Germ-a-Clenz readily cleans dirt off the rind, while killing mold. Simply spray, allow it sit, and wipe off. Or, spray and wipe off immediately. For the mold sensitive Germ-a-Clenz is a boon. Through using it a greater variety of fruit will be tolerated. Plus, Germ-a-Clenz helps remove pesticide residues.

Treatment protocol

Use the Germ-a-Clenz as much as possible to purify the air and cleanse any surface. Use it to destroy mold wherever it is found. A special type of undiluted oregano spice oil, known as Cleaning Oregano, is also available. This may be mixed with soapy water to cleanse and detoxify. It may also be rubbed directly on non-painted, that is woody, surfaces for destroying mold. Take Oreganol oil, five or more drops under the tongue two or three times daily. As an exceptionally potent mold killer take also Oregacyn, the multiple spice extract, one to two capsules twice daily with meals. For stubborn cases take more, like two or three capsules three or four times daily. Strictly curtail the intake of sugar, sweets, chocolate, white bread, white rice, and alcohol. Also, reduce or eliminate the intake of corn products, a major source of molds. Spray any moldy or suspect food with Germ-a-Clenz. It destroys food-borne mold or germs on contact. Use it to also spray the inside of the refrigerator to prevent mold growth. Spray any suspect room and if you have a basement, regularly spray it.

Mold is a major inhabitant of the sinuses. In order to regain optimal health the mold in this region must be destroyed. The Oreganol may be inhaled. Saturate a Q-Tip and place it on the inside of the nose, avoiding the sensitive outer parts. Gently move the Q-Tip up the nose and allow it to remain as long as possible. This will aid in a direct kill of molds in the nose and sinuses. The Oregacyn may also be inhaled, that is the dust. Shake a bottle, open, and inhale the fumes. Add a few drops of Oreganol to a few ounces of salt water and use as a nasal gavage. For tough conditions perform the nasal gavage frequently, like three or four times daily.

Oreganol is a potent mold killer. For eradicating internal mold infections take a few drops of the oil under the tongue twice daily. Also, take the Oregacyn, two capsules twice daily.

Norwalk virus

The Norwalk virus is a kind of flu virus, which attacks primarily the gut. This infection usually occurs in outbreaks, where large groups of people congregate. Outbreaks in the United States are often linked to eating raw or partially cooked shellfish, particularly oysters and clams. Shellfish become contaminated via stool from sick food handlers or from raw sewage. Yet, any food could be contaminated, that is any food, which is contaminated with stool. If the food is poorly washed or not washed, the infection will be spread. The sickness is usually transitory and rarely fatal. The infection can largely be prevented through proper hygiene and through thoroughly washing food. In restaurants there is a protocol to follow to prevent the infection. First, be sure to thoroughly wash all food, especially vegetables and fruit. With seafood, wash thoroughly. In any seafood dish add plenty of spices. Add the contents of a few capsules of OregaMax on or in any seafood dish. When dining, take the OregaMax capsules with and add to food. Drizzle any vegetables or salads with vegetables. For added protection take a few drops of the Oreganol prior to eating.

Parasitic Infections

A major cause of food poisoning and potentially fatal illnesses, parasites are ubiquitous. They may be invisible, however, they are everywhere. Parasitic infections are readily contracted from food, particularly from fresh fruit and vegetables. The parasites reside in dirt and organic residues on the surface. Thorough washing virtually eliminates the risks. However, contaminated water is another primary source of the infection. Worldwide such water is the main source for the infection.

A wide range of parasites can be contracted from fresh fruit and vegetables, including amoebas, cryptosporidium, cyclospora, liver flukes, giardia, hookworms, and roundworms. Unwashed fruit is a major source of the infection in the Third World. However, even in the United States, increasingly, infection is caused from unwashed fruit and vegetables.

Prevention is the key, that is avoiding the infection through proper food handling processes and decontamination. The point is to remove or kill the parasites where they are most vulnerable: outside the body. Once they are ingested, they can often evade the killing actions of medicines by hiding deep in tissues or by invading cells, where they are relatively protected. Parasites are hardy organisms. Every effort must be made to prevent their ingestion.

There are a wide range of parasites which infect humans. These parasites may be divided into categories: worms, amoebas, flukes, and flagellates. Parasites exist in the active or adult form as well as in the larval, cystic, and 'egg' forms. Of the hundreds of species of parasites only a few are notable in terms of human infections, that is exceedingly common. A partial list of the most common human parasites includes:

beef tapeworm

pork tapeworm

fish tapeworm

roundworms

pinworms

hookworms

whipworms

filarial worms

giardia

cryptosporidium

intestinal/liver flukes (from cattle, sheep, goats, pigs, etc.)

blood flukes

amoeba

Blastocystis hominis

Pneumocystis carinii

Skye Weintraub, in her book, *The Parasite Menace*, quotes a disturbing statistic: half of all Americans suffer from at least a minor degree of parasitic infection. Many of these victims are children, who are frequently infected by worms. In American children, she claims, some 55 million suffer a significant infestation. Symptoms of infection by worms in children include poor appetite or ravenous appetite, diarrhea, constipation, itchy skin, itching of the rectum, failure to thrive, dark circles under the eyes, constant sensation of hunger, low energy, agitation, irritability, stomach or abdominal pain, cramps, bed wetting, attention deficit, rambunctious behavior, grinding of the teeth at night, nose picking, weak appearance, pale complexion, nausea, vomiting, and joint pain. Other symptoms commonly seen in adults include irritable bowel syndrome, bloating after eating, blood or mucous in the stools, insomnia, nervousness, open sores on the skin or inside the mouth, excessive nose picking, excessively itchy nose, ravenous appetite or no appetite, restless behavior, insomnia, and impaired immunity.

With parasitic infections prevention is the key. Proper hand washing is critical. Parasites can be easily spread through failing to wash dirt or perhaps fecal residues from the hands. Children notoriously have poor toilet hygiene. Wastes, including feces, become trapped under the nails, and, thus, they reinoculate themselves. Thus, to prevent the spread of these germs the fingernails must be kept short. Routine trimming can largely prevent the transmission of these germs. If the hands are routinely washed and the fingernails kept clipped, the likelihood for transmission is significantly reduced.

Parasites can't be seen. They can get on any object, particularly food. This is where Germ-a-Clenz is invaluable. There is nothing more miserable than a severe parasitic infection. The diarrhea, cramps, pain, and fever are intolerable.

Yet, it all could be prevented, that is with proper hygiene and the strategic use of spice oil sprays. The fact is such infections can be prevented, merely with a bit of care and the use of spice extracts. The fact is the latter kill germs. If proper cleansing procedures are adhered to, along with the intake of a potent multiple spice extract, such as Oregacyn, these aggressive infections can be prevented. The fact is spice extracts obliterate parasites of all types. Worms, amoebas, and protozoans all succumb to their powers. Veterinarians report that such extracts readily purge worms from cats and dogs as well as horses. Thus, for humans Oregacyn can be used as a parasitic purge. Simply take two or more capsules three times daily until the infection is eradicated. With such dosing take a high quality healthy bacterial supplement. Health-Bac is a high grade acidophilus-plus supplement based upon European research: take a heaping teaspoon in warm water at bedtime (i.e. away from the Oregacyn). Also, Intesti-Clenz is a potent antiparasitic, specifically formulated to destroy them. Made with special types of wild-derived spice oils, this is the ideal supplement to add to the protocol, especially for deep-seated infections. In particular, Intesti-Clenz is highly effective in killing worms.

Germ-a-Clenz is instrumental in halting pandemics, whether due to viruses, bacteria, parasites, and/or molds. This is because it attacks the true cause: environmental germs. By attacking and destroying germs in the environment, especially airborne agents, the epidemic or pandemic agent is halted before it can strike. In other words, the germs are killed before they cause harm or death. This is the immeasurable benefit of such a germicidal cleanser. This means that it cleanses filth and chemical residues, while killing germs. It also kills large parasites, including worms, as well as mites. Its filth-cleansing properties are considerable. This makes Germ-a-Clenz the ideal fruit cleanser.

For instance, apples are often waxed. Germ-a-Clenz strips this off, while sterilizing the peel, which makes it of greater value in food handling than even water. Yet, ultimately, Germ-a-Clenz kills the germs which commonly infect humans. Thus, such a substance prevents disease and saves lives.

Treatment protocol

Parasites are difficult to kill. They burrow deeply into tissues, hiding within thick layers of cells and mucous. They may encyst themselves. They also create walls around themselves, that is the typical cysts found in the liver, spleen, lungs, kidney, and/or brain. Megadoses of herbs, the highly pungent aromatic types, are often required. Oregacyn is the ideal parasitic purge. A simple antiparasitic plan is a diet of raw pumpkin seeds, raw honey, along with the Oregacyn. While eating only the aforementioned foods take two Oregacyn three times daily. For difficult cases take also the anti-parasitic formula, Intesti-Clenz, 20 to 40 drops twice daily. Also, take Oregacyn Digestive, which has enzymes that cleanse the bowel and dissolve parasites, three capsules three times daily. Take also as a liver purge, for instance, the highly active GreensFlush, four droppersful twice daily in an ounce or two of extra virgin olive oil. Also, take the Oreganol oil of oregano under the tongue, five to ten drops twice daily. Follow this plan for at least ten days. Once the purge has been achieved, replace the bacteria in the gut with a high-grade healthy bacterial supplement such as Health-Bac. This is sufficient to purge the majority of parasites from the tissues and/or the blood.

Plague

The plague is the common term used throughout the English speaking world for the bacteria responsible for the most deadly epidemic in history. Beginning in 1348 with outbreaks in Florence, Pistoia, and Lucca, the plague quickly spread throughout Europe killing between one-third and one-half of the entire population. This problem was caused mainly by the lack of proper sanitation and thousands of people living in close proximity to one another in the large European cities of the day. Large-scale outbreaks continued intermittently in Europe until 1530, well into the period we consider today as the Renaissance.

Unfortunately, all of the misery and death that accompanied this period could have been easily controlled by working to eliminate a large proportion of the rat population. The presence of rats living with humans in the unsanitary conditions of Medieval European cities proved to be a harbinger of the human destruction to come. The rats, which were afflicted by the bacteria, would be bitten by fleas that would transfer the infection to humans and family pets in the household. This simple mechanism accounts for how nearly half of Europe's population was wiped out between 1348 and 1350.

Nowadays, odds are low for a plague outbreak in the United States. In fact, the last urban outbreak occurred in Los Angeles between 1924 and 1925. While an epidemic is unlikely, this dangerous illness is increasing in frequency, especially in the southwestern states. In fact, the areas that are considered the most heavily affected by the plague are northern New Mexico, northern Arizona, southern Colorado, California, southern Oregon, and far western Nevada. Currently, approximately 10-15 people die from the plague every year in the United States.

Contrary to popular belief, the plague is not a disease for the history books. With reports from the World Health Organization (WHO) of between 1,000 and 3,000 deaths per year, there is still a significant risk for an outbreak. In fact, serious outbreaks have recently occurred in India, Africa, and China. The most effective way to treat this hideous malady, without the side effects of prescription antibiotics, is through the use of all-natural spice extracts.

Plague is caused by the bacterium named Yersinia pestis. As stated previously, this type of bacteria is transmitted to humans via the bites of fleas or by handling infected animals. While this bacterium did create havoc for hundreds of years, the plague is one of the easiest diseases to prevent. This is because with natural antiseptics any potential bite or lesion can be effectively treated immediately. By sterilizing any suspect lesion, the development of the plague may be aborted.

Due to the fact that the plague is caused by bacteria, this means that it can be destroyed by natural spice extracts with antimicrobial activities. Powerful volatile oils from spices can effectively eliminate the "bubonic" or "black" plague. In this era of antibiotic-resistant strains of bacteria it would not be advisable for Yersinia pestis to undergo a metamorphosis that allows it to also become immune. The proper solution in today's dangerous world is the antimicrobial powers of spice extracts, especially Oil of Oreganol P73 and Oregacyn P73. The exothermic reaction created by oil of oregano has been proven by research at Georgetown University Medical Center in Washington, D.C., to effectively eliminate bacteria, as well as fungi and viruses. The plague bacteria readily succumb to the powers of such spice extracts, which are even more potent than the antibiotics traditionally used for this disease.

A recent outbreak (June 2004) highlights the risk. In the state of Colorado alone, 80% of the tested population of prairie dogs carries the plague. In fact, prairie dogs have recently been found dead from bubonic plague. Therefore, in particular, human transmission in the southwestern United States is likely. Pests may readily contract the plague from prairie dogs and transmit it to humans.

The combination of Oregacyn P73, Oil of Oreganol P73, Germ-a-Clenz, and Herbal Bug-X effectively protects the individual from the plague. Regarding the latter, the Herbal Bug-X is ideal. When sprayed on the fur or skin it prevents flea bites, plus it destroys fleas, even those buried in pets' hides. Germ-a-Clenz is another helpful spray which is ideal for sickrooms. In all, this demonstrates the efficacy of oral as well as topical agents for preventing or destroying the disease.

Treatment Protocol

- SuperStrength Oil of Oreganol P73—apply topically to any suspect lesion with liberal quantities. Also take 20 drops under the tongue several times daily.
- Oregacyn P73 Respiratory Support Formula—Take 2 or more capsules three times daily. For extreme cases take 3 capsules four to five times daily.
- OregaMax—Take 4 capsules three times daily.
- GreensFlush—Take 10 drops three times daily under the tongue.
- Herbal Bug-X—Spray on skin and/or fur to kill and/or repel fleas.
- Germ-a-Clenz—spray the air and/or bedding in any sickroom by misting towards the ceiling and allowing to drip downwards as needed.

Optional:

- Purely-C—Take 2 capsules three times daily.
- ZymaClenz—Take 3 capsules three times daily.

Poxviruses

There are hundreds of poxviruses which infect humans and animals. Smallpox is the most well known of these. This disease has been eradicated. However, outbreaks of various animal poxviruses are occurring, for instance, the so-called monkeypox outbreak which is in the United States. This virus is more correctly described as a rodent virus, which occasionally afflicts monkeys. Apparently, it is an African virus, which, interestingly, has recently been studied as a potential biowarfare agent. There would seem to be a coincidence in this. In June 2003 a significant outbreak occurred in the United States. Dozens of individuals were afflicted with a painful, severe illness, manifested blisters and other lesions on the skin and mucous membranes. Other symptoms include fever, sore throat, swollen glands, and rash. The source was infected prairie dogs, which were purchased as pets. Apparently, individuals became infected through close contact with these animals which, in fact, are rodents; scratches or nipping may have also caused infection. Direct contact with prairie dogs was apparently a prerequisite for the infection, although human-to-human has also occurred.

Upon seeing these lesions it is obviously an animal pox. Yet, there is a far greater concern: the plague. In the United States prairie dogs are a primary harbinger of this germ. These animals carry a wide range of diseases. For instance, in New Mexico several outbreaks of plague have occurred in native children. The cause was the habit of native children trapping these rodents for pets.

Smallpox remains a concern, not because of natural outbreaks but, rather, because of the vaccine. This is because the vaccine is made with live virus, and, thus, it readily spreads this infection. In the early 19th and 20th centuries several smallpox outbreaks were attributed directly to vaccination. Truly, the administration of large amounts of commercial live vaccine will result in the return of this dreaded disease. While such vaccination is supported by the government, private medical experts fully question its validity. In 2003 the *New England Journal of Medicine* published an article claiming that such vaccinations bring more danger than benefit. The fact is the reintroduction by the federal government of vaccination with live materials will prove to be one of the greatest public health blunders of all time. Already, a number of people have died as a result of the vaccination. There is another concern: bioweapons. Smallpox could be released into the general public, either by criminals or even the government. The fact is the government has previously sprayed pathogenic germs from planes on unsuspecting citizens. Such spraying has led to sudden death. In one instance a number of people, at least nine, died as a result of the spraying of a germ known as *Serratia*. The fact is the government has no regard for the general public. People are regarded as mere pawns, without rights. Like arial spraying mass vaccinations disseminate germs. The fact is if large numbers of Americans receive the smallpox vaccine outbreaks of this dreaded disease are inevitable.

Treatment protocol

Apply oil of wild oregano on any suspect lesions. Also, take the oil, five or more drops under the tongue as often as possible. For oral lesions make an oregano oil/salt water gargle. In an eight-ounce glass of water add a half teaspoon sea salt plus five drops of the oil. Gargle several times daily. Also, take Oregacyn, two or more capsules three times daily. For strength and energy take a high potency royal jelly capsule, such as the Royal Power, four to six capsules daily. For smallpox cream of tartar has been historically used. Crude red sour grape powder (i.e. Resvital) is a top natural source of this acid: take three capsules twice daily or if using the powder, one teaspoon twice daily. For tough cases take more, like six capsules twice daily and three teaspoons twice daily. For any skin lesions apply the essential oil and propolis-based Oreganol cream. The latter is highly effective at eliminating itching, scabbing, and pustule formation.

SARS

Killer plagues are already afflicting Americans. SARS, which is an abbreviation for severe acute respiratory syndrome, is the latest one. With these plagues people are dying unnecessarily. This is because nature provides a wide range of substances which are useful in reversing these diseases.

Rather than a mere respiratory disease SARS is a systematic killer. The SARS organism attacks virtually all organ systems. It is highly invasive and appears to be an animal virus, possibly from rodents. Apparently, it consists of a combination of bird virus and rodent genes. There may also be a porcine component. This virus aggressively invades human cells, killing them. It also causes internal bleeding and in this respect bears similarity to Ebola. Thus, the name is a misnomer. It should be renamed Rodent-Source Hemorrhagic Plague (RSHP). This is because SARS is manifested by damage to various internal organs, including the liver, spleen, blood cells, kidneys, heart, and, of course, lungs. Hemorrhaging has been documented in all these organs. Thus, SARS truly is a hemorrhagic disease.

Plagues kill many people in the prime of their lives. It is truly a dire crisis, and the consequence is the erosion of the strength of civilization. People are already dying prematurely from AIDS, mutant hospital germs, Lyme, tuberculosis, and West Nile. The medical system is overwhelmed by this crisis. When SARS strikes, how could it handle that?

SARS has already arrived. It is brewing, right here. No one will talk about it, especially at the higher levels. In fact, it is being hushed up. This disease is in the United States, but no one will admit it. People are dying from it. The press is failing to cover it.

In San Francisco, March through April 2003, there was a serious outbreak. In Kaiser Permanante in the Vajello suburb up to 20 people died of an unusual acute respiratory syndrome. Ominously, the symptoms of this infection mimicked the known symptoms of SARS.

This would be the perfect city for the first U. S.-based SARS outbreak: the closest U.S. city geographically to China with an extensive Chinese population. Plus, there is continuous travel of both Orientals and Westerners to and from Asia. It is perfect breeding ground for the outbreak. And this is precisely what happened.

Certain people are highly vulnerable to SARS. People who are over 55 are perhaps most vulnerable, especially those who have received vaccines during adulthood, particularly the hepatitis B and flu vaccines. In fact, vaccine administration is a major risk for developing SARS, especially its life-threatening form. This may account for the high vulnerability for this disease among hospital workers. With the exception of the military they are the most extensively vaccinated of all people. Other individuals with a high vulnerability for developing a potentially fatal type of SARS include people taking multiple drugs, those on antiinflammatory medications, especially the so-called NSAIAs, those who regularly take cortisone, and chemotherapy/radiation patients. The antiinflammatory drugs are particularly dangerous. They directly inhibit the immune response, greatly increasing the risks for SARS infections.

The exact source of the virus is unknown, but it is believed to have originated in rodents, specifically the civet cat, a kind of delicacy in China. From the mongoose family, which is, in fact, a kind of rodent, the Chinese harvest such animals from the wild and sell them in the open market. The meat, as well as saliva and secretions, is infected, and anyone who handles or eats such animals also becomes infected. The WHO recently confirmed that rodent viruses are the likely cause of SARS. What's more, the consumption of rodent flesh, such as the Chinese civet cat, may cause, as well as spread, the disease. I first published about the rodent/civet cat connection to SARS in *The Respiratory Solution*. Now, the Chinese have taken action, confiscating and destroying various rodent-like animals, prohibiting their sale. This has led to an obvious decline in the incidence of SARS.

The SARS virus is a coronavirus, which is from the same family as the virus which causes the common cold. The latter is known as the human coronavirus. A recent study by Microbiotest Labs proved the powers of spice extracts in killing this virus. A test tube was filled with culture material and millions of coronaviruses, in fact, five million per milliliter. Oregacyn was added in a concentration of less than a half percent. Within 20 minutes all traces of the coronavirus were killed. There is no drug available with such a dramatic killing power. Yet, there may be other germs which are causing SARS, that is it may be multi-microbial. This is why Oregacyn, as well as the oil of oregano, is invaluable. Such substances are capable of killing a wide range of germs, in other words, they are universal antiseptics.

Treatment protocol

According to the medical profession SARS is incurable. This is no attempt to propose a cure. However, the fact is spice extracts are potent germicides. Such extracts kill a wide range of viruses. The Oregacyn is particularly valuable. It contains a combination of antiviral spice oils: wild cumin, oregano, sage, and cinnamon. Oil of oregano is also antiviral. A study by Siddiqui published in *Medical Science Research* showed that this oil completely destroyed a wide range of viruses, including the herpes virus.

SARS can be treated, but, usually, the therapy must be aggressive. To kill the virus take Oregacyn, two or more capsules three times daily. For tough conditions take it more frequently, like every hour or two. Also, take oil of wild oregano, i.e. the P73 Oreganol, five or more drops under the tongue several times daily. Rub the oil on the feet, chest, and spine several times daily. For extreme cases use the SuperStrength, ten or more drops under the tongue every hour or even every few minutes.

If you are afflicted with a life-threatening respiratory disorder, have hope. Results will happen; it may be necessary to increase the dosage and frequency. Since they are made from wild spices, which are edible, the Oregacyn and oil of oregano are non-toxic. They can be taken in massive amounts without toxicity. Also, another invaluable technique is to do a foot soak. Using ideally the SuperStrength oil of oregano, pour a half bottle into the bottom of a flat pan; place the feet over this and keep in contact for an hour or longer. Retain the oil residue; use it the following day for further soaking. Consume large amounts of crude raw honey, particularly the wild oregano honey, five or more tablespoons daily. Again, this is far from claiming a cure for SARS. It is merely information regarding natural remedies which dramatically boost the immune system, while providing germ-killing powers.

There is no question that Oregacyn kills germs. This includes the coronavirus, the germ which causes SARS. The fact is as mentioned previously Oregacyn, as well as the Oreganol oil, utterly destroyed a virus of the same family: the human corona- virus. Thus, as a combined therapy the oil under the tongue and the Oregacyn will prove lifesaving. The fact is this potent wild spice oil extract is indispensible, especially in the treatment of life-threatening viral diseases.

Is the real cause known? the role of mites

Seemingly, close contact is a requirement for the spread of SARS. People normally must have a close association: in an airplane with a SARS victim or a doctor or nurse in close contact with a case. Patients give it to their caretakers, while spouses spread it among themselves, and even mothers give it to their infants. Yet, researchers are unclear regarding the exact cause. While a coronavirus has been implicated, definite proof of the full cause is lacking. There may be a yet-to-be discovered mechanism that has been overlooked: the role of mites. These microscopic creatures thrive among human populations as well as near or on animals. In particular, mites thrive near or on hairy animals, including rodents. Mites and similar parasites may readily transmit disease. The role of blood-sucking insects, such as ticks and mosquitoes, in the transmission of disease is overlooked. However, few realize that mites are also blood-suckers and that they carry a wide range of disease causing organisms in their secretions. One of these diseases is hemorrhagic fever. I was alerted to this by a Korean War veteran, who related stories of trench warfare in his division. He described outbreaks of hemorrhagic fever in the troops, which was "more frightening than (fighting) the Chinese". Soldiers watched in horror as their comrades dropped dead, bleeding to death within their internal organs and hemorrhaging from all orifices.

It was quickly discovered that this was no ordinary hemorrhagic fever: it was a type of rat fever. The fever was transmitted not by the rats themselves but by microscopic mites, which fed off the rats. Contaminated with viruses from the rats' blood, these mites burrowed into the skin and/or membranes of their human victims, directly seeding the infection. The result was a fulminant and often fatal fever, which was a primary cause of disease and death in the troops. I interviewed two vets about this. Both said that the fever was far more fearful and deadly than the war itself. There was no cure. However, if clothes or bedding were in contact with a rat, not uncommon in ditch and trench warfare, the clothes were immediately stripped off, doused with gasoline, and burned. According to the vets if direct contact with rats occurred, soldiers would even attempt to burn their hands for fear of the mites. I researched this further. In fact, rats do carry a number of blood-sucking mites.

Difficult as it is to believe, humans are frequently colonized by mites. They readily live in the hair or on the scalp, especially in the hair follicles. They aggressively invade the skin, usually through hair follicles or sebaceous ducts. Mite secretions and feces are potent allergens. This is largely because mites are a filth-creating animal contaminated by potentially deadly secretions and germs.

Mites which infect rats have been implicated in a number of outbreaks of skin rashes. There are also certain types of 'human' mites, which readily infect the hair follicles and sebaceous ducts. Researchers recently pointed to these mites as causing certain disfiguring skin diseases such as acne rosacea, cystic acne, and folliculitis. These mites readily invade the hair follicles on the scalp, face, and chest. It is believed that the majority of individuals have them. They have also been implicated as a cause in balding. Apparently, the mites burrow into the hair follicles in susceptible hosts, choking the blood supply. This results in inflammation of the scalp and/or hair loss.

Close contact with civet cats and other rodents is directly associated with SARS. Animal handlers are at a high risk for developing the disease. This would substantiate a role for blood-sucking mites, which proliferate on these animals. From the animals they could inhabit human skin, as well as hair, injecting the infection.

Mites may be readily killed, that is through the use of edible spice oils. The oils may be taken internally, and they are largely effective through this route. However, they are also highly effective when applied topically. Scalp Clenz is a combination of spice and herbal oils known to kill mites.

Simply apply this oil on the scalp once daily, for instance, at night before bedtime. Cover with a hair net and wash off the next day. Or leave on for 48 hours. Skin Clenz may be used on the face and chest; simply apply once or twice daily. Alternatively, the oil of oregano may also be used, that is the Oreganol olive oil emulsion. These oils are non-toxic and may even be applied to a baby's skin.

Spice oils are also available in a spray. The Germ-a-Clenz is the ideal mite killer, that is for spraying on contaminated surfaces. This is ideal for spraying on bedding, clothes, or even in the hair. What's more, it is convenient to use, since it is emulsified. Thus, it leaves no oily residue. Merely mist on any suspect region. Repeat as needed. This is the ideal spray for spraying pets or pet housings.

Sepsis

This is a debacle of modern medicine. In general sepsis only occurs in the hospital. It is largely due to the overuse of antibiotics as well as surgery. It is defined as overwhelming infection of the blood and internal organs. In other words, it is an infection which is running rampant within the body and which the immune system is unable to contain.

A high percentage of hospitalized patients become septic. In hospitals this is the leading cause of death. Even patients hospitalized for relatively mild disorders may develop it. In fact, such patients may even die from the hospital-acquired infection, while their original problem was routine. Minor surgeries could lead to fatal infections, that is premature or unexpected death.

JAMA reveals an ominous statistic. Some 250,000 Americans die from sepsis yearly, and this is the result of hospitalization as well as the overuse of antibiotics. Thus, these deaths are physician-and hospital-induced. Once the sepsis develops in most instances nothing can be done. Doctors observe helplessly, unable to halt the progression. The patient dies an unmerciful death, all of which was preventable. This is where spice extracts are invaluable. Various wild spice substances, such as the high potency oil of oregano and Oregacyn, obliterate germs, even drug-resistant types. A study at Georgetown University showed that an extract of a number of wild oregano species (the P73 Oreganol) effectively destroyed drug-resistant staph, in fact, as effectively as the most potent antibiotic known: Vancomycin. The oil also destroyed a powerful fungus, Candida albicans, which is notorious for causing hospital-based sepsis. What's more, the Oreganol, as well as the Oregacyn, has been proven in human trials to reverse sepsis:

Case History:

A 14-year-old boy was in a coma from E. coli sepsis. This occurred in Walkerton, Ontario, Canada, the town which was afflicted with sewage- related water contamination. I was called in to give a lecture to the community. One of the mothers attending decided to try the Oreganol on her comatose teenager, by rubbing it on his feet and chest. Within minutes he began responding; within hours he was sitting up in his bed. Incredibly, he was released after 48 hours, with a clean bill of health. Obviously, the Oreganol saved his live.

Treatment protocol

Aromatic spice oils are the key to reversing sepsis. Other than drugs, which are limited, there are no other answers. The oil, preferably the SuperStrength, can be rubbed on the feet as often as possible. Also, add it to juice, water, or milk, as much as can be tolerated. Rub it on the chest and spine as often as necessary. Take also the crude herb, that is the OregaMax: add it to hospital food. Merely open the capsule and add it to meat dishes. For septic patients a combined therapy is required: the oil plus the

Oregacyn. Always give these with food or plenty of fluids, particularly juice. The oil mixes well with milk or meal replacements. The fact is their regular and systematic use could prove lifesaving, even for the desperately ill. The Oregacyn, being ultra-potent, may not be as easily tolerated, especially by the elderly. Initially, use small amounts, like a half capsule mixed in food or honey. Then, as the person gets used to it give a capsule three times daily then two capsules three times daily or more. For extreme situations take the Oreganol aggressively, for instance, ten or twenty drops under the tongue every half hour. Also, give crude raw honey, especially the wild oregano honey, two or more tablespoons several times daily, giving as much as eight ounces daily.

Simian viruses

As freakish as it may seem a high percentage of Americans are infected with simian, that is monkey, viruses. These viruses were introduced into humans, primarily through vaccines. Blood transfusions are another source. An individual who was exposed may have dozens of such viruses in his or her body. This is no minor issue. Simian viruses are among the most potent cancer-inducing agents known.

The primary victims of this incredible pandemic are people born between 1955 and 1964. Such individuals received vaccines tainted with a variety of monkey viruses. The number of different types of monkey viruses is unknown, but it is considerable. The vaccines of this era were contaminated with dozens or even hundreds of viruses, all from animals. The most pathogenic of these were from monkeys.

The reason the vaccines were contaminated is because the viruses were grown in animal cells. This is because viral growth is dependent upon living animal tissue. In other words, to make sufficient vaccine for the populous the virus must be grown in living tissue. Then, it is 'harvested.'

The ideal medium for growing these viruses is living animal cells, notably cells from various mammals. During the 1950s and early 1960s viral research was largely performed on monkeys, and monkey cells were specifically grown for this purpose. Cells were harvested from the organs of these animals and grown in culture. Then, they were infected with the specific viruses for creating vaccines such as measles, mumps, rubella, and polio viruses. These artificially cultivated viruses were then harvested using a crude method that readily allowed contamination. The vaccines produced contained not only the targeted virus but untold numbers of others, whose toxicity was unknown. No attempt was made to purge the vaccines of such contaminants. In fact, it was impossible to do so. Thus, the vaccines were hopelessly contaminated. Anyone who received them became contaminated. Estimates are that some 150 million or more North Americans are infected with monkey viruses. In other words, they have living monkey viruses in their tissues. These viruses are highly aggressive and are known causes of cancer. They are also a major cause of inflammatory, immune, and metabolic disorders, including chronic fatigue syndrome, kidney disease, lupus, eczema, psoriasis, asthma, and fibromyalgia. Attention deficit disorder and autism have also been associated with such infections. What's more, such germs are associated with the onset of a life-threatening, feared disease: cancer.

As early as the 1960s researchers were certain that monkey viruses, notably simian virus 40 (SV40), caused cancer. They had done the experiments. When such viruses, known contaminants of vaccines, were added to normal human cells, the cells turned cancerous. The researchers found that this virus was highly aggressive: in the majority of experiments it effectively converted normal healthy cells into cancer cells.

Thus, the virus was certain to cause cancers in humans. No attempt was made to warn the public of the danger. That proof came later.

John Lear, in his book, *Recombinant DNA*, *The Untold Story*, describes the technique for creating vaccines:

> Vaccines are made by growing virus in tissue culture. As the...vaccines were to be used in humans, cells of the human body would have been the preferred tissue....but in the 1950s the art of tissue culture was still in a primitive state, and the only human cells available for this purpose had been taken from cancer patients. To avoid risk of spreading cancer among humans...viruses were adapted to grow in non-human tissues. And they did grow quite successfully in the cells taken from the kidneys of rhesus monkeys. Ten to a dozen successive generations of this virus were grown in this manner. The ultimate progeny were then given to drug houses for use in the manufacture of vaccines...The safety of all vaccines is an object of constant attention...Various tests were employed in monitoring vaccine quality. One such test...involved the injection of fluid from uninfected rhesus monkey kidney cultures into hamsters. The result was that tumors grew in the hamster. (Then), the same fluid from the uninfected rhesus kidney tissue was injected into the kidney tissues of a different kind of monkey, the African green monkey. Instead of growing as they normally would, the African green monkey cells began to disintegrate. Something that could at first be identified only as a "vacuolating agent" was killing the cells. To find the killer, all the...vaccines were searched for a virus other than (the one it was made for). And every one of them was found to contain a monkey virus that had escaped notice before.

Lear further describes the findings of the polio vaccine, which was given to tens of millions of Americans and Canadians. This vaccine was often given orally, immersed within a sugar cube. A live vaccine, the polio virus was far from the only live organism within it:

> ...the same ban on human tissue culture....had earlier caused the polio vaccines to be grown in kidney tissue of the same monkey. So the polio vaccines now had to be subjected to the scrutiny that the (other vaccines) had just undergone. And their examination showed all the polio vaccines to contain the identical monkey virus..."

Obviously, despite their seemingly prestigious status pharmaceutical houses fail completely when it comes to safety. "Tens of millions" of people took the oral polio vaccine. The majority of these millions were injected with various other vaccines. Incredibly, all such vaccines were experimental: no proof was ever provided of their safety. These vaccines were injected directly into the tissues or in the case of polio vaccine taken orally. No mention was made of possible side effects nor the possibility of contamination. People placed their trust in the medical profession; it portrayed itself as the righteous savior. It was neither trustworthy nor righteous. Rather, it reeked with deceit. It demonstrated only apathy and ignorance, even a total disregard for human health. People placed their trust in the medical system, and instead of health improvement or prevention it gave them nothing but disease and devastation. Regarding the potentially dangerous long-term results of this vaccine no one was given notice, even though the authorities were fully aware of the contamination. The fact is untold thousands of cancers—perhaps millions—were caused by these contaminated vaccines. The administration of these cancer-inducing vaccines marks one of the greatest debacles of human existence, and it was all done for profit. There is no means of determining the extent of the damage. Suffice it to say that the injection of contaminated animal secretions, rife with aggressive, invasive and immunosuppressive viruses, is the greatest cause of death and despair in the human race. This is the vile legacy left by the pharmaceutical cartel, a group which has only one issue in mind: profits.

Tens of millions of North Americans suffer from chronic simian virus infections. The symptoms are vague but significant. Common symptoms include exhaustion, weakness, muscle flaccidity, stiffness of the joints, stiffness of the spine, sluggish immunity, lowered body temperature, tendency to develop tumors or cancers, muscular weakness, flabby muscles, loss of muscle control, seizures, recurrent infections, weakened immune system, skin rashes, psoriasis, eczema, chronic dermatitis, and frequent cold sores or herpes outbreaks, including shingles. Signs include lowered white or red count, swollen liver or spleen, recurrent tumors, and swollen lymph glands. Diseases associated with infection by simian viruses include asthma, autism, attention deficit disorder, psoriasis, eczema, herpes/shingles outbreaks, lupus, multiple sclerosis, ALS, ankylosing spondylitis, fibromyalgia, chronic fatigue syndrome, irritable or inflammatory bowel, Parkinson's disease, brain tumor, and cancer.

This is a highly destructive contaminant. Yet it should be no surprise: it is an African monkey virus, a jungle virus that was never meant to be in the human body. All it can do is cause harm. It is utterly abnormal within the body.

This debacle was fully the consequence of greed and arrogance. People now suffer with pain and disability because of it. The fact is it has caused an immeasurable degree of illness, disease, disability, and death. Often, it renders the victim weak and frail. At a minimum it disables the immune system. What's more, the only hope for recovery is to destroy the organism, which the immune system has failed to eradicate. This requires a stupendous effort, largely through the use of wild or mountain-grown spice extracts. It is terrorism by injection, that is in willing, trusting victims. These are victims who believed in the system, who trusted unwittingly in the status quo. Do not trust the safety of vaccines. The majority of these vaccines are diabolical killers.

Treatment protocol

A fierce effort must be made to purge simian viruses from the tissues. The viruses live in a wide range of tissues, including the bronchial tubes, sinuses, lungs, bloodstream, liver, spleen, spinal cord, and brain. People who are chronically ill are likely victims of such infections.

Again, an intensive effort must be made to eradicate simian viruses. A high percentage of North Americans are infected with such viruses. As late as 1997 the virus was discovered within brain tumor cells of children. This means that contamination of modern vaccines is plausible. Such viruses are deeply rooted, that is they are well established. The immune system has proven to be incapable of eradicating them. Yet, they can be killed, that is through boosting immunity and virus-killing natural medicines. This requires the intake of high doses of Oreganol, the SuperStrength being preferable, under the tongue as well as oral dosing with Oregacyn. Take the oil, five or more drops under the tongue several times daily. Also, rub the oil on the feet and spine as often as possible. It may also be rubbed over the long bones such as the bones of the lower legs and thighs. This causes the oil to gain entrance to the lymphatics, which are extensively contaminated with this virus. Take also the Oregacyn multiple spice capsules, two or more capsules three times daily. This protocol must be followed for a minimum of four months. Beware of counterfeit types of oil of oregano, which are unfit for human consumption. Use only the researched-tested types. Makers of this type include North American Herb & Spice, Vitamin Shoppe, and, in Canada, Vivitas. What's more, do not be enamored by high carvacrol claims: the majority of such claims, upon assay, have been proven false. In contrast, the wild oregano oil by North American Herb & Spice is guaranteed to have a carvacrol content of 54 to 65%, proven by assay.

Staph infection (drug-resistant)

This is a man-made epidemic, secondary to the overuse of antibiotics. Staph is short for *Staphylococcus aureus*. The suffix *coccus* stands for circular shape; this is a round bacteria that grows in clumps. It is highly invasive and is the cause of a wide range of diseases. Staph readily causes infections of the skin, scalp, bones, joints, blood, and internal organs.

Staph is one of the hardiest of all bacteria. It was one of the first to develop resistance to penicillin. Quickly, it mutated, discovering ways to protect itself from such drugs.

After mutating for decades as a result of antibiotics, now it has become a vicious invader, able to damage or kill even young healthy individuals. Every year in the United States and Canada completely healthy children and adults are killed by staph. These are not hospitalized patients. Rather, they are victims of a germ which is an opportunist. Thus, if the conditions are right, it will invade the body and destroy the immune system as well as internal organs, leading to rapid death. There is no predicting who it will attack. Madeline Drexler describes its evil:

> ...a healthy seven-year old girl in Minnesota died from...Staphylococcus aureus infection. Somehow, the bacterium had breached her skin, planted an infection in her right hip, and traveled through her bloodstream to her lungs, overwhelming her body's defenses. Staph is not supposed to kill healthy children. Her doctors were blindsided.

Yet, mutant staph has become far more common since that early era. Now, it is a pandemic, particularly in the United

States, England, and Canada and similar nations, where antibiotic usage is extensive. It is striking even completely healthy people, wreaking havoc on the population with a vengeance. Drug companies, through the overly aggressive use of antibiotics, have created a monster. It is a monster which becomes more powerful every time an antibiotic is prescribed. Only natural cures can halt this monstrosity. People must learn to use such medicines aggressively, that is before it is too late.

Only natural medicines can kill the mutants. A study conducted by Georgetown university proved that drug-resistant staph succumbed specifically to the powers of P73 oil of wild Oreganol. The study, performed in mice, showed that even life-threatening infection could be reversed with natural substances. Even after the infection gained a foothold within the blood and internal organs oil of wild oregano saved lives. Half the infected mice survived, an unheard of result for a natural medicine. Vancomycin, the drug of last result, was also used in the study. It too saved half the lives of laboratory-infected mice. However, the animals taking the drugs were weaker than the Oreganol-treated group. Thus, long-term the Oreganol acted positively upon the immune system, whereas the drug failed to do so.

Treatment protocol

As a potent immune tonic take the oil of wild oregano, five or more drops under the tongue twice daily. Take also Oregacyn, two capsules twice daily. Rub the oil on any suspect lesion as often as necessary. In difficult cases take a large amount of Oregacyn, two or more capsules several times daily (with food). As a potent cleanser and immune tonic, juice antiseptic vegetables such as green onions, yellow onions, radishes, ginger, watercress, and arugula. Add a few drops of oregano oil as a protective agent. Drink a cup daily until the condition is resolved.

Systemic fungus

There are a number of fungi which may infect the body systematically. Many of these fungi cause potentially lethal diseases. Currently, such fungal infections have reached epidemic proportions. There are more than 70,000 known fungi which inhabit the Earth. There are perhaps hundreds of thousands, even millions, which are unknown.

Humans are readily infected by fungi. According to M. Ogholikhan, M.D., in her article, *Recognizing Systemic Fungal Infections* (*Emergency Medicine*, November 2003), in fact, humans are highly susceptible to their infective powers. She writes that in susceptible individuals fungi may not only invade the body but also spread throughout the blood, even to all the organs.

Symptoms of systemic fungal infections may be readily missed. This is because the majority of the symptoms are vague, in fact, common. Typical symptoms include achiness, stiff joints, fever, rapid heartbeat, cough, wheezing, sinus problems, and difficulty breathing, which can be seen in a wide range of diseases. Bizarre skin rashes or lesions may also be noted. A careful history often reveals the true cause: there may be a history of being exposed to the fungus, that is environmentally, or to the risk factors for fungal invasions such as prolonged use of cortisone, steroidal inhalers, antibiotics, as well as the use of chemotherapy drugs and/or radiation therapy. Frequent surgeries, especially if antibiotics are administered, also increase the risks.

In North America there are a number of common systemic fungal infections, which infect tens of millions of people yearly. These infections include blastomycosis, candidiasis, histoplasmosis, coccidiomycosis, sporotrichosis, and cryptococcus. Regardless of the type the consequences are the same: the gradual destruction of the immune system and the body tissues. Fungi are invasive. They are opportunists. Their purpose is to invade and destroy. The definition of a fungus is an organism that lives on dead and decaying material. Thus, if the body is invaded by such organisms it is already in a sickened state.

The growth of systemic fungi is greatly enhanced by invasive medical treatment as well as potent drugs. Cortisone, that is prednisone, greatly encourages fungal invasion, as do potent or broad-spectrum antibiotics. Individuals who take such therapies virtually automatically develop systemic fungus. Symptoms of systemic fungal infections are diverse, including a wide range of digestive disturbances, largely because of the invasive nature of these germs. Mental, joint, and muscular symptoms may also result. The fungi can invade the endocrine glands, leading to a wide range of symptoms as well as diseases, including diabetes. The fact is in all diabetics there is systemic fungal infection. Such infections are also common in other glandular diseases, including hypothyroidism and adrenal insufficiency.

Fungi normally live in the body, causing no major harm. However, when the healthy bacteria, which line the digestive tract, are destroyed—the consequence of antibiotic therapy—the fungi invade, causing a wide range of digestive disturbances. This may account for various vague symptoms such as bloating, intestinal irritation, heartburn, intolerance to certain foods, pain, spasms, cramps, gas, heartburn, difficulty swallowing, diarrhea, constipation, and even hemorrhoids.

Treatment protocol

The treatment for all types of systemic fungal infections is the same: aggressive use of spice oil extracts. Take Oregacyn, the potent triple-spice extract, two or three capsules three times daily. For tough situations take it more often, like four or five times daily. Also, take the Oreganol oil of wild oregano, five to ten drops under the tongue several times daily. For tough cases use the maximum strength variety, five drops under the tongue several times daily. For cleansing fungus and fungal dust from the air use the Germ-a-Clenz; spray once or twice daily. What's more, dietary changes are necessary. Refined sugar must be strictly eliminated. This means halting the consumption of candies, cookies, pastries, doughnuts, soda pop, fruit drinks, fruit pies, and similar foods. If you drink, quit. If you smoke, quit.

Tuberculosis

This is a persistent pandemic, affecting people in every city in the world. The WHO (World Health Organization) estimates that at least one third of the human race, some 2 billion people, suffer from the infection. Not every case is active. Every year an incredibly large number, some two million people, die from this disease. Within the human race TB is a permanent epidemic. It is gradually becoming a common infection, especially in health care workers, hospitalized patients, and people living under crowded conditions.

Tuberculosis is brewing. It is lurching forward systematically, causing a vast human crisis. Russia is the hot-bed for its spread. There, in Russian prisons TB is rampant. Overcrowding has spread the germ, and the overuse of antibiotics has led to the creation of resistant strains. Hundreds of thousands of Russians, both common citizens and prisoners, have developed the infection. What's more, they are infected with a highly resistant strain that defies all medical treatment. These strains could suddenly spread globally, infecting hundreds of millions. In any northern climate TB can readily make a resurgence.

Adequate sunlight is the greatest enemy to this disease. Solar rays are directly toxic to this germ, which indicates that it is more fungal than bacterial. A lack of sunlight allows it to gradually infect the body. Regular sunlight essentially eliminates it from the tissues. Through an unknown mechanism the sunlight penetrates the tissues, ultimately sterilizing the blood of this germ. Apparently, the tubercular germ is sensitive to ultraviolet waves. Dark dreary environments breed this disease. People in northern climates, who live in closed quarters, are particularly vulnerable.

Currently, in Canada in Inuit villages TB is a fulminant epidemic, with as much as 50% of the population affected. This disease is a processed food syndrome. Processed food destroys the immune system, making the individual vulnerable to pathogens. The Inuit who live on a natural diet tend to be immune from it. Thus, it is only in the Westernized Inuit villages, where people live on processed food, where it is epidemic. Yet, in Canada in general there is a growing epidemic. The germ thrives in northern climates, since sunlight destroys it, while a lack of sunlight allows it to breed.

There is seemingly no stopping its onslaught. Hospital workers are becoming increasingly infected. There are a rash of infections developing in doctors, technicians, respiratory therapists, and nurses throughout both the United States and Canada. TB is also emerging in public schools. Currently, a systematic effort to contain it is lacking. Thus, a widespread epidemic is inevitable.

The destruction upon humanity due to TB is unfathomable. Here, it is critical to realize that this is virtually a universal germ, since it infects fully one third of all humans. People aren't born with it: they contract it from the environment or from other humans or animals. In certain parts of the world virtually all residents have it. The fact that one of three people have it attests to its ubiquitous nature. This means it is virtually everywhere, in the water, food, air, and on surfaces. It means that billions of creatures, human and animal, play host to it. It means that untold millions of people, many of whom the individual may come into contact with during his or her lifetime, carry active infections. The fact is the ultimate source for this infection, that is the source that seeds infection, is direct contact between humans. This is the only explanation for the incredibly widespread nature of this disease. Simply put, humans contract TB from each other and to a lesser degree from various animals. This disease is raging throughout human and animal populations. It is only a matter of time before a deadly pandemic resurfaces.

A person with TB usually coughs extensively. Thus, he/she certainly deposits large amounts of the infective bacteria in potentially transmissible regions such as the floor of houses, sidewalks, streets, sinks, etc. Certainly, many of these infective bacteria are killed by environmental factors such as sunlight and exposure. Active germs may be picked up on shoes or by hand and carried back to the home. If on shoes, simply walking on the carpet can disseminate them. A baby playing on the carpet could contract the infection. Waste cans, where sputum-filled Kleenex may be tossed, may also be contaminated. Yet, direct, that is intimate, contact is a more likely source of the spread. Thus, an infected spouse may give it to a mate or perhaps children. Yet, when people have active infections, it may readily be contracted from inanimate objects such as utensils, door knobs, and railings. TB has even been contracted from contaminated books. Obviously, towels and handkerchiefs used by an infected individual readily transmit it. It can even be contracted from contaminated furniture and counters.

The TB bacillus is hardy. If an individual within the family has an active infection, great vigilance is necessary to prevent the spread. The fact is with normal household cleaning methods it is virtually impossible to prevent the spread of this disease.

Airborne spread is another major cause. The sputum may become dried and if pulverized, readily disperses the agent.

Also, air filters can become contaminated with the germ. The tubercular germ breeds here, spreading infection. This is largely how TB is spread on airliners, although direct exposure by sitting next to a coughing, infective individual is a more likely source. The fact is there is today a relatively high risk of developing TB on airliners, especially if active TB carriers are on board. Each year thousands of individuals contract a kind of subclinical TB as a result of airline flying.

Treatment protocol

TB is tough to kill. Therefore, the treatment must be prolonged. However, the oil of wild oregano and the Oregacyn are the ideal killers. This multiple spice extract offers multiple actions against this difficult-to-kill germ. This offers a potent killing effect against this germ. Beware of inexpensive or generic types of oil labeled as Origanum vulgare. These are likely *Thymus capitus*, which is unfit for human consumption. What's more, avoid the aromatherapy grade (not for internal use) types of oil of oregano usually labeled as Origanum vulgare and/or oil of oregano. Unless it says guaranteed wild oregano oil (Mediterranean spice), do not buy it.

For mild to moderate cases take both oil of wild oregano and the Oregacyn, 20 drops under the tongue twice daily; hold it under the tongue as long as possible. Do this for at least six months. Then, follow a maintenance of 10 drops twice daily. Also, take Oregacyn dessicated spice caps, 2 caps twice daily with food, also for a year. Then, take a maintenance dose, one cap twice daily. For severe cases take 20 drops under the tongue four to six times daily; hold it under the tongue as long as possible. Do this for at least six months. Then, follow a maintenance of 20 drops twice daily. Also, take Oregacyn dessicated spice oil capsules, 2 to 3 twice daily with food, also for a year. Then, take a maintenance dose, one capsule twice daily. For extreme cases take the SuperStrength, 20 or more drops under the tongue four to six times daily for at least one year. Then, follow a maintenance of 20 to 50 drops twice daily. Also, take Oregacyn concentrated spice oil caps, 4 to 6 caps three times daily with food, also for a year. Then, take a maintenance dose, one to two caps twice daily. Note: high doses of the Oreganol may destroy the lactobacillus, leading to constipation. To replace these bacteria take Health-Bac, a half teaspoon in warm water at bedtime. If necessary, repeat first thing in the morning.

To neutralize airborne spread use the Germ-a-Clenz. Spray its aromatic essence on any counter or surface where there is concern of contamination. Spray the air and bedding of a sick individual. It may also be used as a throat spray as well as nasal spray.

Other therapies include a high protein diet, whole organic milk (about a pint daily), and organic eggs over easy, soft boiled, or soft poached.

The milk connection is well established. Milk provides a full array of nourishing amino acids plus a wide variety of vitamins. It also provides vitamin D, necessary for the strength of the connective tissues and spine. The spine frequently degenerates in this condition. Only pure organic milk, preferably non-homogenized, is appropriate for this condition. Never use commercial milk, which may be contaminated by bovine growth hormone. The exception is the milk in Canada, which is free of this hormone. Be sure the milk is from herds which are only fed vegetable matter. Organic cottage cheese is an excellent option, that is if milk is poorly tolerated. Eggs are invaluable, because they are highly nourishing, and, therefore, help prevent the wasting which typically develops. Even so, certain people are highly reactive against milk, so this therapy is far from universal. However, one means to reduce the reactivity is to add a few drops of Oreganol in every pint, for instance, five to twenty drops. This helps neutralize any possible noxious or allergenic proteins.

It is also critical to naturally support thyroid and adrenal function: take Thyroset and Royal Power, 4 capsules of each daily. For severe cases take 4 capsules twice daily. These supplements naturally boost hormone function. The Royal Power provides natural steroid hormones—the hormones of royal jelly—for boosting adrenal function.

The oregano oil can also be used as a topical rub. When applied topically, it enters the lymphatic system and, ultimately, enters the lungs as well as blood. On a daily basis rub the SuperStrength oil of oregano on the spine, preferably before bedtime. Also, rub it on the feet in the a.m. and then place the socks on, allowing a natural dosing throughout the day. Repeat the foot rub at night.

Germ-a-Clenz is an ideal agent for preventing the spread of this infection. It helps neutralize this germ before it can spread. Simply spray on any suspicious region or object. Regarding TB a victim's room can be regularly sprayed to decontaminate it. Mist any region which may harbor residues of secretions, like showers, sinks, bathtubs, or beds. Spray all bedding before washing. Also, to halt coughing spray directly into the mouth or on the roof of the mouth. The TB germ may live in the sinuses, and by spraying directly on the roof of the mouth the active ingredients can pass directly into the sinuses. The fact is those with active TB may spread this germ virtually everywhere. Thus, all rooms should be sprayed with Germ-a-Clenz. A single person can infect an entire family, in fact, an entire community.

Tuberculosis is a devastating disease. Every effort must be made to prevent it and to halt its spread. Natural spice extracts are the most powerful natural method to do so.

West Nile virus

This has always been a cause of disease, but never in the Western world. Yet, occasional outbreaks have occurred in

Europe. What's more, prior to the U.S. experience there was an outbreak in Russia. This would appear to be a suspicious event: was this a biowarfare experiment, which had gone awry? Regarding the latter, like the United States, this country is well known for its experiments on encephalitic germs.

Yet, how did the virus get to the Americas? Did the virus suddenly adapt to the Americas, that is through natural transmission? The fact that it is a tropical virus makes this implausible. Or is it a man-made disaster, the release of an engineered virus? Or, did a militarily-produced virus, which was being researched in this country, escape? Or, was it purposely released? All are plausible. However, the evidence points to a man-made virus, which is attested by the CDC's own statement: that animals are being infected by a West Nile-*like* virus. This is the terminology used by both the WHO and the CDC. Neither has come forward with definitive proof that this disease is precisely the same as the one occurring naturally in the Middle East and Africa. No definitive epidemiology has been brought forth. What's more, if it did arise there, is it a genetic freak, the product of genetic engineering, in Israel, Russia, or the United States? The point is West Nile-*like* is not the same as West Nile.

Outbreaks of the disease naturally occur in Africa as well as the Middle East. Recently, there have been outbreaks reported in the Middle East. Here, apparently, it is spread from geese to humans.

It is possible that the Israeli connection accounts for the American outbreak, beginning in New York's large Israeli Jewish population. Yet, no evidence for this direct connection has been provided. It is equally plausible that it has an artificial origin. There is a government bio-lab near the outbreak site: Plum Island. This Level Four facility (the highest is Level Five) has been plagued with accidents, including power outages. Due to safety concerns employees there have gone on strike a number of times. This lab specializes in animal-to-animal and animal-to-human diseases. Thus, various animal viruses, including West Nile-like agents, have been investigated there.

It is a top secret facility. Thus, little is known about its operations. Yet, what is known is that a variety of encephalitis viruses have been investigated, such as the virus which causes West Nile. What else could cause this? If the virus originated in the Jewish community, wouldn't there be a pocket of illness? The original and supposed Jewish source has never been determined. The standard theory is that a mosquito attacked a single Israeli, which resulted in its spread throughout the country. Yet, could a prolonged international epidemic of a germ from subtropical Africa truly spread this way? Could it suddenly become established, even in cold climates, such as Canada, which it has failed to do in nature? What's more, the American virus is more aggressive than the naturally occurring ones. For instance, why would it specifically attack and kill crows, which are notoriously tough? This is utterly different than the African type. Plus, why is it killing a wide range of scavengers: crows, owls, hawks, and eagles? Why does this virus seemingly know no limits, even attacking and infecting cows and wildlife? Why are ducks and geese seemingly immune? American ducks and geese have no immunity to West Nile, so they should be particularly vulnerable. Yet, it is the scavengers which are dying most readily. Obviously, this is a novel disease, not a mere expansion of the African type.

It violates all common sense to believe this is a natural outbreak. It could only occur via an industrial blunder. Or, it could have resulted from a purposeful release, a biological experiment, with Americans as the guinea pigs.

The spread is too bizarre and rapid to be attributed to a natural transmission, like a mosquito transported overseas and then infecting a single New Yorker. Such 'theories' are most likely government propaganda to cover up the true source, that is a biological experiment gone awry. No scientist would regard such a theory seriously, that is the theory that it is an imported virus spread by mosquitoes. Plus, obviously, this type of West Nile virus is exceptionally virulent, far more virulent than any naturally occurring type. No natural type kills such a wide variety of hardy wildlife. Thus, this is certainly a genetically engineered germ.

Treatment protocol

Prevention: use Herbal Bug-X, the edible bug repellent. Rub topically and spray on clothes or skin. Also, take this edible repellent internally, 20 drops once or twice daily under the tongue. Incredibly, through internal consumption under the tongue there is a significant repellent action. The Oreganol also has this action. Avoid the intake of refined sugar, since mosquitoes prefer 'sweet' blood. Eat foods rich in thiamine, which is a mild mosquito repellent. The top sources of this nutrient are liver, egg yolk, red meat, poultry, and fish.

Treatment: in addition to medical care take Oreganol oil of wild oregano, 5 or more drops under the tongue as often as needed; let sit under the tongue as long as possible. Also, take Oregacyn multiple spice extract, two or more capsules twice daily. For severe cases take even larger amounts, for instance, three capsules several times daily with food or large amounts of juice. High doses can kill the lactobacillus. To prevent this eat plenty of yogurt and take the biologically active natural bacterial supplement, that is the Health-Bac, a heaping teaspoon in warm water at night before bedtime. Make a raw honey and vinegar tonic; take a quarter cup twice daily. Also, drink fresh citrus juice, about a quart daily.

Whooping cough (pertussis)

Like measles this is resurging in the Western world. Incredibly, the primary victims are the vaccinated. Apparently, immunization directly introduces a form of this germ, which chronically establishes itself in the body. It is a mutated form, so in most instances it fails to elicit immediate symptoms. Because of the suppressed immune system secondary to the immunizations the bacteria take a foothold, leading to active infection. Non-vaccinated people can also get it, usually from exposure to immunosuppressed vaccinated individuals.

Whooping cough is caused by a bacteria, which infects the respiratory tract. This disease is also known medically as pertussis. The bacteria directly invade the lining of the respiratory tract, where it causes significant irritation and inflammation, resulting in the distinctive whooping-like noise upon expiration. This noise frightens people. Yet, it is important to note that this disease is rarely fatal.

Throughout America whooping cough is making a significant comeback, especially among children and adolescents. Vaccination offers little or no protection. The fact is there have been a number of outbreaks of this infection in vaccinated populations. Entire families, not just children, have contracted it, despite vaccination. This modern type can prove fatal, yet, the germ can be readily destroyed through the powers of wild oregano. Wild spice extracts kill this germ. In the event of active infections the results are often dramatic.

Treatment protocol

For severe cases take Oregacyn, which is a potent antispasmodic agent: one to two capsules three to four times daily. Also, take the oil of wild oregano, two or more drops under the tongue as often as needed. This is not a difficult germ to kill. It merely takes persistence. Raw honey is invaluable, a teaspoon or tablespoon as often as necessary. Use a truly wild and raw honey, where the bees are never fed sugar. With most commercial honeys the bees are fed sugar. To order wild non-sugar fed honey call 1-800-243-5242. What's more, the oil can be rubbed on the feet and chest as often as needed. As a result of the oil and Oregacyn therapy this condition will be rapidly cured.

Vaccine overload

Gulf War Syndrome is a debacle beyond comprehension. Men and women who supposedly gave their lives for their country are the victims of a brutal experiment. This syndrome is directly caused by vaccines.

Gulf War Syndrome is definitive evidence of the unmerciful toxicity of modern vaccinations. Garth Nicholson, Ph.D., has fully demonstrated that this syndrome is largely due to vaccinations. A diabolical "therapy," vaccines are the cause of incalculable misery and devastation. This is because they are contaminated.

No one who is thinking clearly would allow contaminants to be injected in his/her body. Yet, with vaccines people do so unthinkingly. This is because there is a certain degree of trust for the public official, the typical attitude of: "If the government endorses it, it must be safe: no one would purposely harm us." Yet, this bizarre practice is far from safe, since it introduces into the body a wide range of contaminants, including highly dangerous germs known as stealth pathogens. These pathogens originate from a wide range of animals, including chimpanzees and monkeys.

It was Professor Malcolm Hooper, England's chief science adviser to the veterans association, who said that without question "troops are clearly suffering from vaccine overload." He clearly determined that the massive inoculations given to servicemen entering the Gulf War are, in fact, a primary cause of disease. His term overload is highly descriptive. The vaccines fully overwhelmed the immune system, in fact causing immunological diseases. According to British investigators, who are holding hearings regarding vaccine overload, symptoms such as bizarre rashes, eczema, mental disturbances, and lung disorders are directly tied to vaccines. In other words, the men and women of Western armies were "poisoned" in the line of duty.

Vaccines are toxic. They contain definite toxins in the form of preservatives, antibiotics, and germicides. What's more, vaccines greatly burden the immune system, fully overwhelming it. The fact is rather than preventing infections they are a primary cause. Outbreaks of polio, whooping cough, diptheria, and measles—even leukemia—have been directly tied to inoculations. So have infections by a host of unexpected germs: contaminants. It is fully established that vaccines are extensively contaminated with known, as well as unknown, germs. This is the legacy of these injections, that is the creation of novel diseases never before known. How can a cure also cause disease? The fact is evidence is lacking that vaccines aid the health of the populace. What is certain is that people have been sickened and many have died as a result of modern-day inoculations.

The toxicity of vaccines has been confirmed by Polish and Russian investigators. These researchers have determined a direct association with certain cancers, notably lymphoma and leukemia, and vaccinations. The researchers had determined that vaccines—even those which are supposedly sterilized—introduce germs, which attack the immune system. The germs directly invade the critical immune organs, including the thymus, lymph nodes, and bone marrow. Here, they cause massive damage, particularly to the nuclear material. This ultimately leads to cancer. Thus, it is the vaccine viruses, which, in fact, incite cancer, where without such exposure it may never have occurred. This is demonstrated by the fact that cancer tissue from a wide range of unusual cancers, some of which had, prior to the introduction of vaccines, never occurred, contains the vaccine viruses. The vaccine-introduced viruses apparently take over the genetic material of the immune cells, as well as internal organs, causing damage to the genes and, ultimately, inducing cancer. Is this anything except the most diabolical and evil deed known? It is all this and more. Bolgnesi, publishing in *Cancer Research*, found a direct link: that vaccines introduce viruses, which cause leukemia. Polish investigators confirmed this, showing that smallpox vaccination led to leukemia. Here, they determined that viruses and other germs introduced by the vaccines attack lymphoid tissues found in the bone marrow, causing them to over-grow. This is the beginning of cancer. In the United States a similar debacle was observed with the more common vaccines such as the MMR (measles, mumps, and rubella). These too have been associated with cancers, notably lymphoma. Researchers discovered an ominous fact: that in lymphoma victims the lymph nodes in the intestines contain the MMR viruses. The viruses apparently attach to tumor activating sites on the cells, converting them to cancer cells. Thus, instead of contracting the measles, a curable and temporary condition, the vaccine recipients receive a cancer-causing virus, which may prove incurable. Incredibly, the very therapy which people place their trust in to prevent disease is, in fact, causing deadly conditions. Again, childhood vaccinations cause cancers: there is no doubt about it.

Yet, the fact that the substrate, that is the liquid, used to form vaccines is carcinogenic has been long known. According to Lear in his book, *Recombinant DNA*, since the late 1950s it has been known that vaccines cause cancer. This was merely covered up, that is by business interests. However, the government's claim was that information about the cancer-causing effects of vaccines would be withheld to avoid causing "public panic." Thus, the federal government itself, as well as the drug companies, which made and sold the vaccine, was well aware that vaccines would cause human cancers. They knew that the policy they instituted would lead to human harm. Yet, they did nothing to rectify it.

In Poland researchers concluded that modern vaccines are, in fact, "tumorigenic." What an incredible ordeal, that is that people trust in a system—the system of modern medicine—only to gain precisely the opposite of what they seek: ill health, even premature death.

It was Michelle Carbone, Ph.D., Loyola University, who first exposed the debacle of modern vaccines. He found live ape viruses growing in human tumor cells as well as diseased human cells. The source of the virus: the oral polio vaccine.

The exposure of the contamination of these vaccines was met with skepticism and derision. Carbone was ridiculed and almost lost his job. Yet, such contamination was already proven. It was just that no one had previously proved it was causing human disease. What Carbone had done was show that without doubt the vaccines are poisonous and are responsible for a vast degree of human disability and disease. One issue is certain: the polio vaccine has resulted in a wide range of diseases, including specific kinds of cancers, notably lung, bone, and brain tumors. Benign tumors of these regions in children also may be vaccine-induced. This certainly gives credence to the belief that vaccines cause a greater degree of harm than good. Carbone's discovery makes the latter statement hard to refute. Since his work was published it has been confirmed by some 60 other studies. The latest study determined an ominous finding: that SV40—the infamous stealth-like monkey virus, which originally contaminated vaccines in the 1950s—secretes into the tissues one of the most potent carcinogens known. Thus, the number of cancers caused by this vaccine contaminant are beyond count.

Similar contamination occurs as a result of modern vaccines, for instance, the meningitis, influenza, and hepatitis B vaccinations. In fact, because such vaccines are genetically engineered they may prove even more dangerous. This is because these vaccines introduce a new variable: human-made toxins and human-created stealth pathogens.

The wanton damage caused by modern vaccines is largely due to a new government policy: a lack of testing for toxic effects plus "immunization" by the government against lawsuits. In 1996 the *Journal of Infectious Diseases* reported that due to the high cost of testing new vaccines the modern vaccines would merely be injected into the unsuspecting public. The people would serve as the test population. Then, a wait-and-see approach would be taken, to determine if there was any long-term toxicity. Incredibly, money would be earned by the pharmaceutical houses without any risk for liability. Lobbyists would be paid-in-full. This while people would suffer from uncountable symptoms and diseases. This is unheard of in this country, since the United States is based on litigious claims. It amounts to governmental sequestering of murderers. This is because without question modern vaccines have resulted in sudden death, that is obvious deaths, which could only be caused by such agents. Yet, with all other industries or people there is culpability and liability, but not so with vaccine makers? Under what guise could such a policy be formed? A supposed need for security or public safety? The fact is this policy has usurped public safety and security.

The epidemic introduced by the early polio vaccine is undeniable. As a result of this vaccine millions of Americans have been infected with various animal viruses, many of which are cancer-causing. Yet, today's polio vaccine is far from safe. Stocks which supposedly have been purged of the offending agents have apparently not been purged. According to the *San Francisco Chronicle* in 1970 long after the vaccine had been declared free of the germ, surgeons found the brain of a two-year-old to be "riddled with SV40". The victim, Mark Moreno, is still alive and he lives as an invalid with his mother. Interestingly, according to Mrs. Moreno in 1968 her son had received the oral polio vaccine, which as had been proven by analysis was the cause of the tumor. Yet, even more alarming is the case of Alexander Horwin, who died in 2000 as a result of an SV40-contaminated brain tumor. In 1997 he had received the oral polio vaccine. Yet, the dilemma is simply explained by Carbone, who states categorically that the "SV40 virus is carcinogenic (in humans)." What's more, this is a powerful virus, which aggressively kills human cells. Thus, at all costs it must be purged from the tissues, that is before it causes irreversible disease.

As early as the 1960s researchers knew that this virus not only destroys living cells but it also causes cancers. Yet, no effort was made to warn the public, in fact, a cover-up was initiated. The fact is the government knew that the vaccine was dangerous yet failed to recall it. More than a million doses of the contaminated vaccine were in the hands of doctors or in hospitals: all were administered. Nor did officials notify the medical profession about the types of cancers caused by the vaccine. Incredibly, scientists employed by the pharmaceutical giant, Merck, fully explained this attitude, saying that government officials were warned that any negative information would jeopardize the vaccination program. What a vile deed it was. Thus, rather than a requirement for the protection of public health vaccines are a public health disaster. They are administered because they are money-making, not because of any proven health benefit.

The science behind vaccines is shoddy. There is little if any proof of benefit. Consider the 2003 flu vaccine and the agent it was used against: the Fujian flu. The CDC flatly said that the vaccine offered no guaranteed protection against such a flu strain. Yet, people were urged, in fact, coerced, to get it. This is an unscientific approach. In fact, it violates the principles of science, which are to have an accurate basis for any claim. Thus, the insistence upon getting the 2003 flu vaccine was a business—even political—decision, not a medical, that is scientific, one.

Vaccination is big business. Could vested interests be interfering with the public interest, fully willing to put people at risk, merely for profits? This is seemingly the only answer regarding their use, since there is little if any proof that they work or that they are safe.

Treatment protocol

For people who have received multiple vaccines a combination approach is necessary: detoxification plus the killing of any bizarre germs. It is critical to purge from the body both microbes as well as toxins such as formaldehyde, aluminum salts, and mercurial compounds. All are highly toxic to the immune system. To purge the toxins take GreensFlush drops, the wild greens extract, five droppersful in an ounce or two of extra virgin olive oil. Also, take the LivaClenz Formula, two or three capsules with full meals twice daily. This will help aggressively purge the liver of toxic components. The Oreganol P73 Juice is invaluable: an ounce twice daily is ideal. The Juice is also invaluable for purging microbial contaminants, especially those which attack the nervous system. It is also anti-proliferative. In the event of serious vaccine toxicity increase the dosage to two or more ounces twice daily. In extreme toxicity as much as a bottle per day may be consumed. One other benefit is that the Juice is an excellent diuretic, plus it helps strengthen the heart muscle. To decontaminate germs and genetic contaminants take the triple spice formula, Oregacyn, two or more capsules twice daily. Take also the oil, that is the Oreganol, five to ten drops under the tongue twice daily. For tough cases increase the dose to twenty or more drops twice daily. For extreme exhaustion add the unprocessed royal jelly, that is the Royal Power, four capsules once or twice daily.

In extreme cases topical treatment with the oil may prove invaluable. Using the SuperStrength Oreganol rub over the large bones vigorously, for instance, the tibia and femur. Also, rub the oil up the spine. Afterwards, scrub with a dry brush or washcloth until reddened, but do not abrase. Repeat daily or every other day, that is until significant improvement is noted. Also, in such cases high doses of Oregacyn may be necessary: three capsules three times daily. Always take the Oregacyn with food or juice. Also, on such high doses be sure to replace the natural bacteria, since high dose Oregacyn may kill even the normal flora. As a potent natural way to replace these bacteria take Health-Bac natural acidophilus supplement, a heaping teaspoon in warm water at night before bedtime. Do not despair. Oregacyn, the Juice, and the oil can detoxify even the most extreme degree of vaccine toxicity. The only variable is how much to take. Plus, the key is to be persistent. Failures are usually the result of too short a course of therapy, that is the failure to take a large enough amount for a sufficient period. Thus, it may be necessary to purge the virus over a series of months, even years.

There is no toxicity with wild oregano products. This is an edible spice, which is free of side effects. It may be readily taken with any medication. The fact is as a 'side-effect' it reduces the need for medication. Wild oregano even aids in the removal of drug-related toxins from the body.

Chapter 4
Staying Powerful

The human race is besieged with infectious diseases. The food supply is unsafe and the air is foul. Closed spaces are readily contaminated. People vigorously spread germs among themselves. Even relatively healthy people are becoming infected. The sick, frail, and elderly readily succumb. Thus, all people are at risk for disabling infections and even life-threatening ones. It is time for people to fight using the most powerful defense possible.

Spice extracts offer such power. Test tube studies prove that wild spice extracts, such as the highly potent Oregacyn (sold by physicians under the name Oregacillin), obliterate pathogens, even drug-resistant germs. This has also been duplicated in humans. The fact is viral levels in humans plummet as a result of the ingestion of such agents. The oil of oregano (P73 Oreganol) is also potent. However, the Oregacyn is the most powerful of all and, therefore, is ideal for life-threatening epidemics. Combined therapy provides the best results, the oil under the tongue and the Oregacyn by mouth.

The other option is to have a powerful immune system, however, this alone is insufficient. It is the combination which is necessary: the potent germ-killers and a strong immune system.

Regarding building the immune system it takes effort to achieve this. People damage their immune systems unknowingly. The objective of this chapter is to make clear what are these damaging factors and how to avoid them. Plus, foods, vitamins, and herbs which boost immunity will be described. It is critical to keep the immune system in the most optimal state possible.

Global infections, which afflict all levels and nations of humanity, already exist. Every year throughout the world people die prematurely by the millions, all due to infectious diseases. Africans are dying by the millions due to a wide range of infections, including AIDS, hepatitis, dysentery, tuberculosis, malaria, drug-resistant germs, and chronic immune deficiencies. Medicine offers few if any solutions. In fact, it has worsened the dilemma, rather, it has caused it. Even so, the worst is yet to come. Soon pandemics will strike, which will afflict the general population globally. Those who are unprepared could suddenly die. Thus, a well designed plan is essential.

For global infections it is crucial to have a plan. The plan must be well thought out as well as scientifically based. Plus, it must be implemented well in advance. Thus, in order to survive the future epidemics, in order to be guaranteed the ability to live through unexpected, as well as existing plagues, epidemics of infectious diseases, it is necessary to know what to do in advance.

When the pandemic strikes, it will be too late. The SARS and West Nile debacles, as well as AIDS, have proven that. Such pandemics have infiltrated the population, becoming epidemics long before they could be controlled. Without a plan people are left to panic, that is if disaster/disease strikes. The plan listed in this book, that is the various protocols, provides a sense of security. It gives the individual a sense of strength, that is to realize that much can be done and to know precisely what to do. It is to realize that there is much which can be done to improve health as well as to preserve it. There is another plan that is necessary. Yet, what a severe consequence there will be if there is a lack of a plan. Germs have a battle plan. What's more, if bizarre germs are synthesized, such as those produced for biowarfare, obviously, there is a plan for such agents. Yet, do humans have a plan for combatting such killer germs? The fact is people must have a plan, that is if the intention is to survive.

Before a pandemic strikes the plan must be known. In other words, it must exist in advance. It must also be implemented well in advance. The individual must know exactly what he/she will do to such a degree that the reaction is natural. Plus, any required therapies or medicines must be available—in advance. When the pandemic strikes, it will be too late. The SARS and West Nile debacles, as well as AIDS, have proven that. Without a plan people are left to panic, that is if disaster strikes. A solid plan makes you feel strong about yourself and even stronger about your life, that is how to preserve it. There is another plan that is necessary. This is the divine plan.

People are mortal. No one lives forever. Ultimately, all people die, becoming transformed to what is essentially an unknown consequence. This requires planning as well. That is for ultimate success death and its consequences must also be prepared for. This too will assist the individual in the ultimate security: the proper understanding of the next world.

Regardless of how secure or healthy a person is there is a definite reality: life is short. What's more, it may suddenly end: shattered by an accident, destroyed by a disease. This is far from an attempt to create fright. It is merely a fact of life. In other words, there is no escaping it. People die. Then, there is a transition. All people transit; all issues change. There is an essence, which disappears upon death. The soul is real. Science proves it.

There is evidence that all is under a mighty control. People may either believe in this or refuse it. However, a person could refuse any idea, even a truth. A person's hostility or refusal fails to give evidence against an issue. Certain facts remain undeniable. When a person dies, an essence is liberated. Scientists prove this essence weighs as much as seven ounces. That essence escapes and proceeds to another realm: it is the life force, which is immortal.

The immortality of the soul is difficult to deny, while, certainly, the physical body is mortal. It is a loss of the most enormous extreme to fail to prepare for this fact, that is that there is an immortal essence in every human. Where will the human go? That is a critical consideration. A person's future holds in the balance: the future in the presence of the highest power: almighty God Himself. So, each person must consider: what preparation is needed to please the almighty maker, who made every individual in his/her unique form?

Each person is truly different, fully unique from all others: in personality, physique, and attitude—and in beliefs. To think of God and, in fact, love Him, is the highest level a soul can reach. This is the ideal to pursue. This is because no one exists due to his/her own devices. All that exists is created. A creative being, obviously, made humans, while also providing all that is required: food to eat, water to drink, shelter, and warmth. Thus, who else is there to love—who else is there to be grateful to—other than the creator of all, the true provider, the giver of mercy?

Each person is a creature of God. Only He knows the true personality as well as the inner self. He alone knows the internal workings of the mind and body, even the inner thoughts. What's more, only He can give warning, directly to each person—in each person's heart.

Recent evidence proves that people who have a purpose, in fact, who believe in the powers of God, are healthier psychologically than nonbelievers. Why deny the inevitable? No one lives forever. Why suffer in fear or confusion? All that is necessary is to reach out in love and gratitude to the almighty One who is always ready and ever hearing for His creation.

Pandemics create fear, in fact, fear of death. This has become evident as a result of the recent (2003-2004) so-called Fujian flu pandemic. People reacted due to all manner of emotional issues: fear, guilt, and 'responsibility.' Yet, the fear of sudden death was perhaps the greatest motive. People begin to realize their mortality. Yet, the key is to never fear it. Rather, the solution is to deal with it, that is rationally. Consider the basis of existence. In other words, consider the true origins of humans. Human beings could never have arisen accidentally. They are too complex. Obviously, because each is unique, as well as highly complicated—each must be a created being. Obviously, no one merely appears by chance. Such a sophisticated being, so refined in structure and function, certainly has a Source. What's more, it makes sense that all arise from this same Source, and all must ultimately return to it. That Source is a power beyond human comprehension but which, incredibly, seemingly cares for every human being. Thus, truly, is there anything to fear?

The purpose of life is to serve a higher purpose: this is what people of faith believe. Perhaps there is reason to fear, that is if the individual fails to serve on a high plane. Yet, it is never too late to do so. All that is needed is to beg the presence of God, who is eager to hear His servants. Furthermore, He is eager to be within them. Studies show that people who feel the need for the divine being and who, in fact, worship Him, are at far greater peace than those who refuse such a concept. As a result, such individuals are far healthier, both physically and psychologically, than those who refuse to accept His presence.

Or, is such a being a product of a higher, more organized power? In other words, is such a being here for a purpose? It makes sense that this is true, since each person is unique and each has his or her own special skills. Each has special talents. Those talents must be exercised for the true purpose to be achieved. They are talents which would appear to be divinely ordained. Yet, who decided on those talents? Who made the concept itself: that of talent and ability? Who made each person utterly unique, that is in those very talents?

There can be no doubt about it: each person is unique. Consider a human family: brothers or sisters? Are they anything but utterly different? Consider their physical features as well as their attitudes and talents: truly each is unique. Down to their fingertips and within the deepest recesses of their hearts each is completely different. Certainly, mere chance evolution could never result in such a wide variety of humanity, with each person being different not only physically but also emotionally and spiritually.

Having a purpose creates productivity. It creates change. It produces positive results. To have a purpose is to accept a higher role. In order to accept that purpose a person should do everything possible to protect his or her self, that is in order to fulfill that preordained role. Each person can accomplish many great achievements. Yet, this is only a minor component of a human being's purpose. There is a far grander objective: the pleasure of almighty God. People who believe in such a concept are, in fact, the most physically healthy of all. Perhaps this is because such individuals are in tune with a higher person, even a higher energy. Psychologists have proven that belief in a supreme being, as well as the active service for such a being, creates health improvement. This is because, certainly, such a belief is in tune with the universe itself. The fact is the greatest advancement is to become a success not only in this life but also in the future one, that is the life where the soul resides: the afterlife.

To fight infection the body has to be in optimal condition. To survive a global pandemic the person must be in top shape. Even then if the germ is potent enough there is no guarantee of safety. Yet, having a strong immune system unburdened by toxins is the most reliable guarantee. This can be largely achieved by a strong spiritual constitution: the lack of fear and panic. Without the understanding of the purpose of life, there will be a degree of panic, especially regarding illness and death.

When severe infections strike, the immune system wages a war to save the person's life. This is precisely the time when each person must remain in the strongest state of health possible. In this instance no one can afford to pollute the immune system, that is through faulty dietary habits. A key method for achieving this is to avoid the substances which deplete or damage immunity. This is precisely the purpose of this section.

For optimal immunity a person's habits must be assessed. This is particularly true of dietary habits, yet there are other factors. The mental condition greatly impacts immunity, as does the spiritual tendency. Recently, researchers determined that belief in a higher purpose, in fact, belief in a supreme being, leads to a stronger, healthier immune system. Perhaps the immune system is in tune with a higher power, which guides it in a way that is unknown. The point is fighting or resisting nature leads to immune suppression. The fact is atheists die prematurely, that is compared to believers.

There are few natural compounds which suppress immunity. The fact is the majority of natural substances, such as herbs, spices, and healthy foods, bolster immunity. The majority of the immune toxins listed in this section are synthetic chemicals or adulterated foods. Even so, there are a few natural substances of note, for instance, mycotoxins. Such toxins are made by molds and are among the most dangerous immune toxins known. Mycotoxins are associated with a wide range of diseases, including arthritis, diabetes, cancer, and heart disease.

The danger of immune toxins

There are a number of substances in the typical Western diet which poison the immune system. Most people are unaware that their own dietary habits are hurting them. The fact is they are unaware that such habits could cause their premature demise. To stay healthy it is important to maintain a strong immune system. Thus, it is crucial to remove all immune toxins from the diet and/or lifestyle. The first step to having vital health is to avoid creating illness.

People frequently create their own illnesses, perhaps unwittingly and even with reckless abandon. Thus, they assault themselves with all manner of noxious substances, which greatly diminishes health. They inflict a kind of self-destruction upon their immune systems, gradually diminishing their health power.

The immune system can be readily poisoned. To keep it strong it is necessary to know what poisons it and avoid such poisons. Incredibly, among the most potent of all immune toxins are common foods and food additives. This section pinpoints the most common toxins, which are extensively consumed by Westerners. As part of the epidemic-cure plan strictly avoid all immune toxins.

Nitrates

Added primarily to meat products, nitrates are a major immune toxin. The toxicity has been known since the inception of these additives in the early 1900s. Then, scientists warned of the severe toxicity of nitrates to human cells. The fact is it is this chemical that greatly depresses the immune system. According to Kedar Prasad, Ph.D., upon ingestion nitrates are converted by the body into nitrosamines, the most potent carcinogens known. It is a carcinogen because it significantly depresses the immune system. I will never forget the last time I ate nitrate-contaminated food: a beef stick. After eating it I developed a massive cold sore. At that moment I decided never again to eat such foods. Avoid nitrated meats at all costs. They are a significant cause of cancer as well as heart disease. Heavy consumption can even precipitate heart attacks. In children the regular consumption of such meats can cause a wide range of disorders, including mental conditions, behavioral disorders, heart disease, and even cancer. Plus, they depress immune function, increasing the likelihood of sudden infections. Thus, in order to remain infection-free it is crucial to avoid nitrated meats. Meats containing nitrates include ham, bacon, sausage, bologna, hot dogs, pastrami, salami, and pepperoni. These are unhealthy meats. There is no reason to eat them. For more information regarding the toxicity of such substances see the book, *How to Eat Right and Live Longer* (Dr. Cass Ingram, Knowledge House Publishers).

Hydrogenated oils

One of the most vile food additives ever synthesized, hydrogenated oils are a travesty of modern civilization. Such oils are unfit for human consumption. Calling such oils a food additive is even misleading. The fact is hydrogenated oils are known carcinogens. Plus, they depress immunity, making the body vulnerable to microbial invasion. The fact is hydrogenated and partially hydrogenated oils corrupt all body tissues, because they are essentially plasticized fats. This means that, while they are used by the cells as a part of their membranes, they fail to nourish them and, rather, distort them. Researchers have proven that hydrogenated oils fully damage human cells by distorting their membranes.

Hydrogenated oils interfere with immunity through a variety of mechanisms. As previously mentioned they directly poison cell membranes. This has an exceptionally negative effect upon white blood cells, which rely upon their normally fluid membranes to attack and consume microbes. As a result of hydrogenated, that is synthetically hardened, fats the white blood cells become sluggish. Their membranes become stiff. Thus, they are unable to properly perform their functions.

There are hundreds of foods which contain these oils. A partial list of foods laced with such oils includes doughnuts, pastries, granola bars, breakfast bars, pop-tarts, waffles, cupcakes, pies, cakes, crackers, cookies, microwave popcorn, commercial peanut butter, cinnamon rolls, French fries, Tater Tots, hash browns, batter-fried food, breaded fish, tortilla chips, corn chips, imitation cheese, muffins, commercial bread/buns, bagels, tacos, creamed soups, creamed vegetables, TV dinners, commercial cereals, and potato chips. Avoid such foods at all costs. Truly, foods containing hydrogenated and partially hydrogenated oils are unfit for human consumption. Do not be misled. Such oils are potent carcinogens. These oils, which are artificial, are responsible for an untold degree of human harm. Thus, they should be prohibited from the food supply.

Refined vegetable oils

Most people are familiar with the toxicity of artificially hardened fats such as partially hydrogenated and hydrogenated oils. However, few are aware that the typical liquid vegetable oils are equally toxic. These oils include commercial corn, safflower, sunflower seed, peanut, and canola oils. Regarding the latter this is a common additive in health food stores. This fails to make it healthy: it is still a refined vegetable oil. These oils are heated excessively, causing their structure to be distorted. This makes them toxic, and, thus, when they are ingested, they greatly disrupt the immune system. Such oils disrupt the membranes of white blood cells, interfering with their ability to search and destroy microbes. The toxicity of heated, refined vegetable oils is great and is dependent upon the degree of the heating. The fact is hot, refined vegetable oils, such as the oils found in deep-fried and snack foods, are among the most potent cancer-causing agents known. In contrast, pure butter and extra virgin olive oil, that is if not heated excessively, aid immune health. These truly natural oils strengthen the immune cells, so that they can more readily destroy invaders. Pure coconut oil is also an immune aid. It contains a special fatty acid known to destroy bacteria and viruses, that is lauric acid. What's more, coconut oil can be heated to reasonably high temperatures, that is without toxic damage. Use these oils instead of commercial/refined vegetable oils. As a result, the immune system will be benefit greatly. Yet, any heated oil must be used in moderation.

Refined sugar

A major source of disease, refined sugar may be the most commonly consumed immune disrupting agent known. Virtually all Westerners consume it, largely as an additive of processed foods. The extensive consumption of refined sugar is a rather recent phenomenon. As early as the 1840s in North America sugar consumption was nil. Then, sugar salesmen gave out sugar packets, specifically to cause addiction. They were highly successful. Americans developed a ravenous appetite for the substance. The sugar addiction era had begun.

Today, the per capita sugar consumption exceeds 150 pounds per person. That amounts to approximately 15 ten-pound bags of this poison a year, more than a ten-pound bag per month. That is a catastrophically large amount. Imagine it: the average person eats per month at least an entire ten pound bag of this useless 'food.' Plus, since this is an average, incredibly, there are individuals who eat perhaps three ten pound bags: a whopping thirty pounds of sugar per month. Such sugar consumption thoroughly destroys the body, ultimately causing organ failure. In fact, refined sugar causes its own specific disease: diabetes.

Professor Yudkin, former professor emeritus at London's Queens Hospital, showed an even more diabolical link: the role of sugar in heart disease. In fact, he proved that in the Western world prior to the introduction of refined sugar there was little or no heart disease. As sugar consumption rose so did the incidence of heart disease, stroke, and high blood pressure.

Sugar destroys the heart and arteries. The fact is yearly thousands of deaths due to heart attacks, strokes, blood clots, and high blood pressure crises are directly due to sugar consumption. Recent data also correlates sugar with the growth of cancer. Is there any other option except to curb, even eliminate, its intake?

There is no nutritional value in refined sugar. In fact, it destroys nutrients. Specifically, it depletes chromium, magnesium, zinc, copper, potassium, thiamine, niacin, pantothenic acid, folic acid, and biotin. The fact is the regular consumption of refined sugar leads to a severe deficiency of these nutrients. What's more, these sugar calories amount to the replacement of healthy nutrient-bearing calories with utterly empty ones. This is why Americans are so unhealthy as well as obese.

Iron contamination: the role of fortified (white) bread products

Inorganic iron, the type added to foods, disrupts immune function. It contaminates the internal organs, causing iron toxicity. This type of iron is inexpensive, and this is why it is used by the food processors. It is, nutritionally, of only minimal value. In fact, its toxicity greatly outweighs any benefit.

Synthetic iron pollutes the body. It is, after all, little more than dissolved iron metal. Thus, since it is a heavy metal it creates a burden of toxicity on the tissues. Research proves that this metallic iron readily accumulates in the tissues; the body has a difficult time dealing with it. If intake is continuous, it ultimately accumulates in excess, particularly in the liver, heart, bone marrow, spleen, and brain. Here, it causes extensive damage, predisposing the individual to heart disease, cancer, and brain disorders.

Synthetic iron is difficult to digest and absorb. In nature iron is specially processed, that is by plant and animal cells. This renders it into a non-toxic absorbable form. Always get your iron from natural sources. High quality natural sources include red meat, liver, spinach, raisins, prunes, crude red grape powder, wild oregano herb (i.e. OregaMax capsules), parsley, cumin, sardines, and egg yolks. OregaMax, which is the pure unprocessed wild herb, helps naturally build blood. Organic eggs are an excellent source of iron, and liver is an excellent iron-rich meat. Another is organic spinach leaves drizzled with lemon and topped with crude red grape powder (i.e. Resvital). The Resvital is naturally rich in iron and can take the place of iron pills. The lemon and crude red grape aid in the absorption of iron. Never take synthetic iron pills.

White bread and flour products

There is no nutritional value in white flour products. This food is extensively refined. The vitality factors which are needed for strong immunity, the natural oils, vitamins, and minerals as found in the bran and germ, are removed and/or destroyed. What's more, the flour is bleached and adulterated. Thus, instead of building the immune system it damages it. The old Wonder Bread signs from the 1960s were ultimately torn down as dictated by the government as false advertising. This was because scientific studies proved that rather than "building the body" white bread destroys it. These studies found that animals fed on white bread fared so poorly that feeding them mere cardboard sustained them better. Thus, incredibly, white bread, utterly adulterated, chemically treated, and refined, is a physiological poison, which should at all costs be avoided. Rather than offering nutritional value it destroys nutrients, ultimately putting the individual at risk for chronic diseases. White bread and, in fact, all white flour products, are unfit for human consumption.

All commercial white flour products are fortified with iron. This is the same synthetic iron mentioned previously. This iron accumulates in the body, causing toxicity.

Artificial flavors and colors

These substances are entirely synthetic. Most are made from coal tar or petroleum residues. Most artificial colors and flavors are known carcinogens. This was fully established as early as the 1920s, when government regulators ignored research in favor of the chemical companies. Thus, despite warnings from researchers and consumer groups these cancer-causing dyes were approved for human use.

In order to keep the immune system in ideal condition avoid the intake of such substances. These purely synthetic— and toxic—substances are found in hundreds of commercial foods. They should never be consumed, since they are highly toxic to the immune system. These dyes directly suppress the function of the white blood cells and in high enough doses kill them. Foods containing artificial colors and/or flavors include commercial ice cream, candies, cakes, pies, cookies, soft drinks, alcoholic beverages, fruit drinks, pickles and pickle relish, candy bars, colored commercial cereals, frost-sticks, slushes, and gum.

Synthetic, that is coal tar, dyes must be strictly avoided. People have no idea regarding the degree of toxicity of these substances. The fact is they are among the most potent carcinogens known. No food should contain them.

The body is highly vulnerable to the toxicity of artificial colors. These substances, which are largely derived from coal tar, are virtually impossible to decontaminate. Thus, they poison the cells, causing damage which is difficult to reverse. The only logical solution is to avoid their intake. Read all labels carefully. If any food contains artificial colors, FDC dyes, or similar substances, do not buy it. Strictly avoid the consumption of synthetic dyes. As a result, an overall improvement in health will occur.

Alcohol

This is one of the most potent immune depressants known. Few people realize it, but alcohol greatly damages the immune system. It significantly increases the risks for degenerative diseases and cancer. It denudes the mucous membranes, allowing microbes to assault these membranes. Alcohol is a major nutritional toxin, depleting a plethora of nutrients. Nutrients readily destroyed by this substance include all B-vitamins, vitamin C, vitamin A, essential fatty acids, and amino acids. It also aggressively depletes minerals, especially zinc and selenium, the latter being directly needed by the immune system. Alcohol aggressively destroys magnesium, a crucial heart and joint mineral. This may explain the high vulnerability of alcoholics to heart disease, high blood pressure, stroke, and bone loss as well as fractures.

People are often misled about the supposed health benefits of alcohol. Yet, while certain alcoholic beverages contain a degree of nutrients, for instance, wine and beer, there are no overall positive benefits to the immune system. To keep the immune system in optimal condition alcoholic beverages must be avoided.

Vaccines

People should know the facts about vaccines before taking them. The side effects of vaccines are rarely publicized. So, people merely assume they are safe and undergo vaccination without hesitation. They have no idea regarding their toxicity. They simply presume them to be safe. "Why would the authorities harm us?" they think. "Why would the government allow it if it is dangerous?" they consider. Or, they simply never consider any issue and blindly trust in the system. Or, they fear the consequences of defying the system, and, thus, are willing to risk all. Yet, the majority of people are simply unaware of the vile nature of these injections and, therefore, subject themselves to undue harm.

The fact is vaccines are among the most noxious and dangerous of all medical procedures. The effects are only rarely noticed, that is acutely. It is the long-term consequences which are vile. Vaccines depress the immune system. Notice what is happening with SARS. Hospital workers are the primary victims. These are the people who get the most vaccines. In fact, they regularly receive them.

It has been long known that vaccines depress the immune system. When they were first introduced in the early 1900s many physicians regarded them as vile. They knew they caused serious side effects. Then, there was no vaccine lobby to cover it up. The fact is between 1900 and the early 1940s many doctors refused to give them to patients out of fear of serious side effects. Dr. L. Bush describes the extent of this debacle in his book, *Common Sense Health*. Published in the 1930s Bush describes vaccines as not a scientific procedure but a mere fad. He notes that many medical procedures in vogue are eventually proven to be faulty, in fact, dangerous. He places vaccines in this category.

The problem with vaccines, he notes, is the unknown. They represent the introduction of foreign elements, protein, and even germs—even pus—into a person's blood. The reaction which might occur in the recipients' blood is unpredictable. Yes, there may be an increase in resistance against the specific disease particles which are injected. Yet, at what price? Bush notes that physicians observed even in that early era an ominous consequence: the loss of resistance against all other diseases. To quote Bush:

> An instance of this occurred in the late war. After being vaccinated for smallpox, typhoid, and paratyphoid, we found the soldiers, who should have been the healthiest specimens in the nation, seemed to lack their immunity to such childhood diseases as mumps, measles, and whooping cough. Hundreds of soldiers were in the hospitals suffering from these infections. Most people were to develop immunity to these diseases as they become adults. Apparently, nowhere near the percentage of adults outside the army developed these troubles as within it, and I question if in any previous war any such condition existed. The outdoor life and training in the army should raise one's resistance rather than lower it; yet, the mortality in the influenza epidemic seemed to be fully as high in the army as in the civilian population. These facts would cast suspicion upon the vaccines used with all of the soldiers while the civilian population made use of them to only a slight extent.

Bush makes another astounding observation. He describes a seemingly definite increase in cancer incidence secondary to vaccinations. Other authors prior to him described the similar findings. Cancer, he notes, became increasingly common by the 1930s, and this is precisely when vaccines became mainstream. Before cancer became an epidemic, the only vaccine commonly administered was smallpox. Cancer incidence can be directly correlated with the administration of multiple vaccines such as diphtheria, tetanus, measles, mumps, and numerous others. This is largely because certain germs instigate cancer, and vaccines introduce these. During that era the quality control of vaccines was poor. Bush makes a connection between the chronic immune irritation from the injection of various vaccine-related toxins and germs and the onset of cancer. What's more, the propensity for vaccines to incite cancer is dependent upon their source. If such vaccines are harvested from animals ridden with cancer, then the cancer may be given to the previously cancer-free recipient. In other words, the vaccines may directly inject cancer materials or, as has been discovered more recently; cancer-causing germs. Incredibly, even merely introducing the foreign blood from an animal which has no active cancer but has a genetic propensity for it is sufficient to incite this disease. In other words, there is a powerful component in the vaccine, which can control cells. It is a component which can convert a healthy system into a cancerous one. Today these are known as cancer-causing viruses, that is viruses which convert normal cells to cancerous ones. Bush categorically recommends against taking vaccines, that is unless they can be proven to be safe over the long term. Such proof, he claims, has never been provided; unless such vaccines can be proven categorically free of the danger of transmitting either cancer susceptibility or actual infections—or outright causing cancer—they should be prohibited.

Patients, claims Dr. Bush, suffer chronic ill health from vaccines. Usually, they are unaware that vaccines are the cause. Incredibly, he concludes, mandatory vaccination should be halted; let those who truly believe in it take it at their own risk. The proof will be in the long term result. If vaccines are truly great, surely, he proposes the dissenters will be wiped out. Surely, all that will be left will be the vaccinated. Today, this theory is failing to hold up. It is the vaccinated people who are dying easily, and the greater the number of vaccines which are received, the weaker and more vulnerable the individual is to fulminant disease as well as sudden death. Thus, as described by Bush it is not the people who fail to get vaccinated that are a menace to society. Rather, it is the immunologically weakened and vulnerable vaccinated people, who develop and even spread disease, that is who are the source of chronic immune deficiency. The fact is they not only develop serious diseases but also spread them. This is demonstrated by the 1918 pandemic, which killed 40 to 60 million people, in other words, more people than could be counted. The source of the spread was vaccinated troops, particularly Americans, who were extensively vaccinated. Yet, this noxious effect of vaccines was recently confirmed: in 2004 a CNN poll determined that people who were vaccinated were twice as likely to develop the flu as those who avoided the vaccination. What's more, also in 2004 as described by Susan Doland, M.D., of Denver's Children's Hospital, in a study of over 1000 vaccinated individuals the flu vaccine offered no measurable benefit compared to those failing to receive the vaccination.

There is little if any scientific proof demonstrating a value for vaccines. By avoiding toxic and contaminated vaccines, the individual preserves his/her health. As a result, he/she becomes an energetic, productive individual, with greater resistance against the plagues which are destroying humankind. I have helped certain mothers avoid vaccinating their children. As a result, these children are among the most immunologically competent children in this society, in fact, such children are far stronger physically than their vaccinated counterparts.

There is an important issue regarding vaccines that is often neglected. It is virtually impossible to sterilize them. They are contaminated with an uncountable array of germs. Severe contamination is rife. Since the late 1990s dozens of vaccine labs have been closed by the FDA due to contamination concerns. A wide range of unknown and bizarre germs have been found to contaminate commercial vaccines, including viruses, mycoplasmas, TB-like germs, and molds. Thus, vaccines are essentially a microbial cocktail. Billions of germs may be injected through a single vaccine. Many of these germs are unknown, plus, certainly, their effect on the body is unknown. Thus, in the 1930s the premise of many physicians was that vaccines are truly experimental, that is their long term effects are both unproven and uncertain, which has been confirmed by today's findings. What's more, they exhibit known toxicity. Dr. Bush closes this subject with a basic concept. He says the diseases which the vaccines supposedly prevent are rare. Is it worth the risk, he queries, to suffer long-term consequences, to, in fact, contract a vaccine-induced disease, merely to prevent a rarity, like diphtheria, whooping cough, tetanus, or mumps? Vaccines are animal byproducts, and there is no guarantee that the animals used to harvest them are disease-free. The fact is the animal materials used in the production of vaccines carry a wide range of disease-producing germs, which will weaken the immune system and, in fact, cause unmerciful diseases. The majority of these germs will never be known. They are stealth in nature.

Reversing the toxicity: the power of spice oils

Spice oils are the Mediterranean mountains' wild treasures. Few people realize that many of the common spices grow in mountainous regions. Thus, they develop in a relatively pure environment, uncontaminated by the hand of man.

Spice oils are perhaps the most powerful of all natural medicines. The individual needs power to overcome the degree of toxicity, which leads to disease. A toxic body is readily contaminated by germs. What's more, when the body is overloaded with toxins, its ability to fight off germs, as well as recover from infection, is compromised. Slow recovery is a sign of tissue overload, that is with noxious chemicals and vaccine residues. It is the spice oils alone which offer the power to purge such toxicity. This is because in addition to their ability to stimulate tissue cleansing they also kill noxious germs, which poison the body.

All germs secrete poisons. Such poisons intoxicate the tissues, ultimately leading to disease. Spice oil extracts, such as Oreganol and Oregacyn, obliterate germs. This eases the toxicity upon the human body, allowing the body to heal/recover. By killing the germs the tissue levels of such toxins dramatically decline.

Today, there is no guarantee in relying upon the immune system to ward off serious infections. The individual needs every boost and aid possible. It is the spice oils which offer such aid in a highly effective and dependable manner. Research proves that of all herbs it is only spice oils which dependably destroy a wide range of pathogens and, which, therefore, can be relied upon in an epidemic. The fact is spice oil extracts, particularly those made from spices, that is the Oregacyn and Oreganol, are veritable natural antibiotics: more so, since such extracts destroy not merely bacteria: they destroy the entire gamut of germs. Plus, they are free of serious side effects. In contrast, as described by the *Journal of the American Medical Association* antibiotics alone are ultimately responsible for tens of thousands of deaths yearly. These deaths are caused by the development of mutant bacteria, which destroy the tissue and organs. No such effect is seen with Oregacyn or Oreganol. In fact, human evaluation has demonstrated that the regular, even long term, intake of such extracts, in fact, improves the organs and other tissue. No toxic effects are noted.

Therapeutic methods

There is no benefit in exposing the dangers of pandemics without also demonstrating the solutions. Incredibly, nature provides definite answers. Yet, the synthetic world, the purely man-made approach, fails to provide them. During 2003-2004 this became clearly evident. Then, the flu pandemic proved resistant to any medicine or vaccine. In fact, the vaccine utterly failed to protect against it. Thus, people lived in fright, panicking and waiting in long lines to get a vaccine, which was of no consequence.

Yet, why such incredible fear? The fact is people fear death to such a degree that they fall vulnerable to scare tactics and, thus, they panic. Because of fear and panic rash decisions are made. People rush to get vaccines and antibiotics, which are useless, in fact, counterproductive.

There is need for deeper thinking, that is to understand the purpose for personal existence. Is mere pleasure and entertainment the only purpose for life, or is there a higher goal for existence? Now, people are realizing that each human should do all that is possible to seek excellent health, physically, emotionally, mentally, and spiritually. Yet, the great bastion of power in terms of health is in the physical. If the body is physically sound, virtually anything may be accomplished. If it is weak, little if anything can be achieved. However, the physical and spiritual are interconnected. A diseased spirit quickly results in a diseased body.

Dozens of remedies of nature are provided. All produce solid results. Most are food based. The proper diet is also included. Foods, spices, and herbs all possess curative properties. Simply try these natural medicines. Alter the diet as recommended. You will be impressed with the results.

Lymphatic therapy

When a person is ill, often, there is little desire to ingest food. This is an instinctive response of the body. All the body's energy is directed towards reversing the infection. All energy is reserved for immune activities. Instinctively, the body tells us to avoid solid food and, in fact, at best to sip on beverages and/or broths. While the gut rebels against solid food, there is another means of administering the medicine: the skin. This reinforces the immense value of spice oils such as the high mountain, highly pungent Oreganol. Such oils can deliver therapeutic actions through the skin, because spice oils are readily absorbed through the skin barrier.

It is the lymphatic system which vigorously absorbs spice oils. The fact is an ideal therapy during an infection crisis, especially epidemic flu, is to do a lymphatic scrub. Too, the old-fashioned mustard poultice over the chest acts on the lymphatics. The poultice is placed over the breastbone, the site of the thymus. Thus, the spicy pack activates this gland, greatly facilitating the immune response. In a similar way Oreganol scrubbing activates the immune components, boosting the immune system's ability to destroy germs. The SuperStrength is the most effective form for such scrubbing.

How to do the scrub

Simply rub oil of wild oregano (olive oil emulsion) vigorously into the skin, starting with the bottom of the feet or lower legs and working up to the top of the thigh. This delivers the oil directly in the lower part of the lymphatic tree, and from there it is disseminated throughout the lymphatic system, including all the lymph nodes and even bone marrow. Also, rub it up the spine, again in an upward fashion. Then, using a dry washcloth buff the skin. This procedure accelerates the absorption of the oil through the skin. The buffing improves the local blood flow to the skin, which, again, speeds the entry of the oil. This is an invigorating procedure and even the most desperately ill individual usually notices a benefit.

Dental dosing

The teeth harbor a wide range of noxious germs. Such germs are capable of disrupting immune function, even causing disease. The teeth also contain a great number of nerve reflexes, which play a monumental role in tissue balance. The fact is a diseased tooth disrupts the nerve and muscular balance in the entire body. Plus, such a tooth causes severe immune suppression.

In severe infections treatment of the teeth, that is the destruction of any pathogens which are infecting the teeth, tooth sockets, and/or gums, can greatly ease the disorder. Such a treatment releases the immune system of the burden of infection. The results are often dramatic: a rapid cure of the infection.

The method of treatment is simple. Line the gums with the oregano oil twice daily. The ideal time is first thing in the morning and right before bedtime. Or, at night saturate a piece of cotton with the oil, and pack it against the upper reaches of the gum line. Also, the oil may be used during toothbrushing, a drop or two on the brush. The Juice may be used as a mouth wash. Using a half ounce hold in mouth for a few minutes, gargle, and swallow. This helps increase the strength of the gums as well as all other oral tissues.

The crude herb: tissue builder

Crude wild oregano, that is the unprocessed wild herb, has its own unique healing attributes that are impossible to achieve with the oil. This is because the wild herb contains a wide range of natural chemicals helpful in maintaining health.

Wild oregano is a top source of a plethora of nutrients, particularly minerals. It is a superb source of naturally occurring calcium and magnesium as well as zinc. All such minerals are required to keep the body in optimal health. Yet, these minerals are also needed by the immune system, and this is particularly true of zinc. This mineral is needed to activate the thymus gland to make thymic hormones. It is also needed by the white blood cells for the destruction of pathogens. Zinc greatly aids immunity. OregaMax, that is the maximum strength wild herb, provides a type of zinc that is well utilized by the body.

The high calcium and magnesium content is also critical. This is because such minerals are needed for bone density as well as muscle contractions. When the bones and muscles become weak, which is a consequence of calcium and magnesium deficiencies, the immune system also becomes weak. The individual becomes susceptible to various infections. The bone marrow is a key immune organ. It degenerates as a result of a lack of key minerals. Thus, by taking the wild oregano-based OregaMax, the individual adds another dimension: a powerful musculoskeletal system, which is an impediment to disease.

OregaMax is also ideal for bone density, in other words, it is capable of reversing that dreaded disease: osteoporosis. However, to do so large doses are necessary such as 6 or more capsules daily. For severe cases of osteoporosis 8 to 12 capsules daily may be necessary. This is far from a difficulty. The OregaMax has a superb taste. It may be added to any stir fry, soup, or salad. It is ideal for sprinkling on applesauce, cottage cheese, oatmeal, and even peanut butter.

Crossing the blood-brain barrier: the Origanum waters (Oreganol P73 Juice)

Oreganol P73 Juice is, in fact, the essence of the wild herb. Such an essence, the product of steam distillation, is known as hydrosols. It is the hydrosols which are rich in oxygenated compounds. This gives them attributes distinguished from the oil.

Perhaps its greatest benefit relates to its actions on the brain. Here, it is a potent healing agent, in fact, preservative. Today, there is great danger against it: stealth viruses, which attack and infect brain tissue. The Oreganol P73 Juice acts against such viruses. It is also an invaluable tonic for the gut. For all types of intestinal disorders it proves invaluable. Its actions on these tissues is readily explained: the Juice provides potent forms of natural oxygen in the form of oxygenated compounds.

Ideal for diseases associated with low oxygen the oregano juice can prove lifesaving. It is an indispensible aid for conditions such as asthma, bronchitis, emphysema, irritable bowel syndrome, Crohn's disease, ulcerative colitis, intestinal parasites, mental disorders, Alzheimer's disease, Parkinson's disease, and obstructive lung failure. All such diseases have an element in common: they are all associated with low oxygen levels in the tissues.

The juice is an invaluable supplement for neurological damage. Because it is water soluble, it readily crosses all barriers. Thus, brain tissue can benefit from its powers immediately. With salt and water it may also be used as a nasal gavage. Simply dilute the juice two to one with water and add a few sprinklings of sea salt. Dissolve and inhale, keeping the head tilted backwards.

Germ-killing foods

There are relatively few foods capable of killing germs. Yet, all hot or tangy foods have this potential. If such hot foods and spices killed human cells, none of us would be alive. Thus, the heat-power they contain seems to be preferentially directed against microbes. Consider oregano, the most powerful food-derived germ killer. The fact that it is from food tells all: it is completely safe.

Everyone eats oregano. Obviously, it can't harm humans or human cells. However, in high amounts it kills virtually every germ it is tested against. According to a study published by Cornell University other foods and spices that are universal killers include onions, garlic, and allspice.

In medicine the fact that foods or food extracts have germ-killing properties is relatively unknown. Yet, there is a plethora of research proving this. Plus, there is personal experience: people who have used foods as medicines, including for killing germs. Consider the garlic necklaces, which in the early 1900s mothers placed on their children, or mustard plasters, which mothers packed on the children's' chests. There must have been a reason for this. The fact is mothers knew that such natural substances both protected against infection as well as reduced the symptoms, that is the course of the disease.

Onions

It was onion rations which supposedly gave Alexander the Great's troops strength to carry out their conquests. The fact is onions have been relied upon for physical and immune power for thousands of years.

Raw onions offer the most power. True, there is the odor issue. However, when dealing with life-threatening infections, such considerations must be secondary. Onions kill germs outright. All germs thus far tested against onions have succumbed.

Onions are high in certain nutrients, including vitamin C and potassium. To get the vitamin C they must be eaten raw. From a germ killing point of view yellow onions are the most powerful, followed by white and red onions. Vidalia onions contain relatively little killing power.

No one can dispute the microbial killing power of onions. Tests routinely prove their potent actions. The fact that onions kill virtually every germ known proves that they are a reliable pandemic cure. Plus, their availability proves their value. Onions can be found everywhere: in every city and store in the country. Always keep a good stock of onions in the home. You never know when you might need them.

Garlic

Caustic and smelly, this is, for obvious reasons, a true microbe antagonist. It both kills germs outright as well as inhibits their growth. It also strengthens immune defenses, aiding in the immune system's ability to hunt and destroy invaders.

Garlic's use as a germ-killer is memorial. In ancient Egypt it was applied to treat septic wounds. In the 17th century it was administered to combat the plague. In the 19th century Louis Pasteur determined in lab studies that garlic decimated germs. No germ tested against it survived. In the 20th century during the first world war British physicians used it to cure septic wounds and gangrene. Most people have heard the early American folk use: mothers who used garlic necklaces, apparently successfully, during the 1918 flu pandemic.

When eaten raw, garlic is caustic. It is also malodorous, in fact, offensive. Yet, in this state it is an effective germicide. It is somewhat less effective when cooked, yet it is still active. As the early American experience proves even the fumes of garlic are germicidal. It may be cooked in hot water and the fumes inhaled. It may be crushed and the resulting fumes inhaled.

Recent research proves that garlic kills germs. When placed in germ-filled test tubes or petri dishes along with inoculations, few microbes survive. One study showed that garlic is even more powerful than potent antibiotics. In a study to determine its ability to kill fungi garlic proved superior to the aggressive antifungal agent, amphotericin B. Scientists have recently determined that raw garlic in particular can kill even relatively tough bacteria, the kinds that antibiotics are often incapable of killing. The bacteria which succumbed to its broad-spectrum killing powers included salmonella, staph, strep, proteus, E. coli, and mycobacteria.

Ginger

The modern world owes ginger to traders of the Middle Ages: the Muslims of Islamic Spain. During the 9th through 12th centuries they popularized ginger, which they brought from the Orient, as an additive to spicy and sweet dishes. They also popularized it as a potent and versatile medicine. Soon, Europeans began trading vigorously for this spice, both as food and medicine.

In ancient India ginger was relied upon for virtually any disease, especially digestive disorders and arthritis. The fact is ginger, a real vital food, is a universal tonic. Regardless of the illness it has positive benefits. This is because ginger stimulates the very processes which keep the body vital: proper digestion and metabolism as well as strong or balanced immunity.

Ginger has powerful "pharmaceutical" properties. It is anti-infective, anti-parasitic, and antiinflammatory. It is also antispasmodic, which means it fights intestinal or stomach spasms.

Ginger must be relied upon in the event of a pandemic. It should be added to all cooking. It should be routinely added to hot teas and cold beverages. Fresh ginger is the most potent type, although dried ginger may also be valuable. Don't rely on the typical spice ginger, the ground type in the supermarket. For dry ginger try oriental or specialty stores.

They may have freshly dried whole ginger, which can be ground at home. This is nearly as potent as the fresh. A special kind of ginger is available, which can be added to any food or beverage. It is a highly concentrated form, so all of ginger's invaluable properties are concentrated in a few easy-to-consume drops. This Oil of Ginger is far more convenient than fresh ginger, plus it is far more potent. To order call 1-800-243-5242 or in Canada 1-800-668-4559.

Vinegar

This remedy was first popularized during the seventh century by the Prophet Muhammad. He recommended its use extensively, describing it as an invaluable condiment. This was fresh vinegar, made without chemicals or additives. He dispensed it as a general tonic. This is precisely the modern finding. Vinegar has a tonic effect upon the gut, greatly strengthening the intestinal and stomach membranes, while enhancing the secretion of digestive juices.

Vinegar is a mild antiseptic. Because of its acidic pH, it inhibits the growth of a wide range of germs, including yeasts. Molds and yeasts thrive in a basic pH; acidic substances inhibit their growth. True, occasionally, molds grow in vinegar, causing a visible cloudiness. Yet, when this acidic substance is consumed, it, in fact, aids in the prevention of microbial overgrowth. Even so, if vinegar contains visible mold, do not use it. If it is regularly consumed with food, it offers an additional benefit. According to Jarvis the most strategic use of vinegar for prevention is when eating in restaurants. He claims that vinegar is a guaranteed preventive against food poisoning. To avoid food poisoning be sure to consume vinegar with every restaurant meal. He claims this formula will prevent untold cases of food poisoning. However, there is a caveat: the vinegar must be taken with the meal, not hours later.

Crude raw honey

It was again the Prophet Muhammad to whom humankind owes this remedy. He firmly established raw honey as an invaluable medicine. This is because the revelation he represented, that is the Qur'an, named it so. Here, it is described as both food and medicine, that is for the benefit of humankind.

As a medicine honey was relatively unknown in Europe. Thus, it was this man who introduced it to the Western world

Crude raw honey, directly from the hive without processing, is a potent cure. In nature it is unprocessed, and that is what keeps the bees healthy. Thus, for humans to gain benefits they too must eat it in an unprocessed state.

Crude raw honey is highly effective for a wide range of digestive complaints, including upset stomach, irritable bowel, diarrhea, and constipation. It is also a general aid to digestion. People with sluggish digestion often benefit from a teaspoon or more daily, taken in the morning before breakfast.

When applied to skin, raw honey has been shown to kill germs as well as speed healing. This completely natural substance, which is non-toxic, has been shown to reverse a number of diseases, including kidney disorders, weak heart or heart failure, septic wounds, intestinal infection, constipation, and burns. This is a God-blessed remedy. The bees make it, and humans gain the benefit. It is is even useful on burns, even the most severe types, for preventing infection and speeding healing. In burn wards physicians in England use it to speed the healing of burns and to prevent scar formation.

The *Journal of Pediatrics*, as well as the *British Journal of Surgery,* reported dramatic findings. The latter, in an article entitled "Clinical Observations on the Wound Healing Properties of Honey", demonstrated a cure rate higher than any medicine. A group of 58 individuals with disastrous wound infections were completely cured through honey applications. Only one patient failed to be cured. That is a 98% cure rate. The wounds had previously been treated with surgery and antibiotics. The *Journal of Pediatrics* showed that even commercial honey has value. In this study infants with diarrhea were treated with honey versus the typical synthetic sugar solution. Only the honey stopped the diarrhea. A Russian experience is similar. In a man who suffered from a huge infective boil several inches across, surgery had failed. Raw honey packs were applied. In a matter of weeks complete healing was achieved. Incredibly, in Germany raw dark forest honeys have been used in sanitariums as a fasting cure. German physicians even cured diabetes on raw honey fasts. Recently, diabetics have reported that a special medicinal honey, mountain derived, is medicinal: the wild oregano honey. Such honey is well tolerated and fails to cause any diabetic crisis. However, do not attempt a wild oregano honey or dark forest honey fast, that is unless under a doctor's care. Even so, instead of orange juice or candy for a blood sugar boost the wild oregano honey would be infinitely safer, plus it is medicinal.

A truly raw honey is unheated, extracted with a centrifuge. It is also minimally filtered and, thus, contains virtually all its native medicinal properties. What's more, such honeys are completely natural in their source: they are derived from plant substances collected by bees, in other words, the bees feed exclusively on the products of nature. In contrast, commercial beekeepers feed their bees sugar syrup as a supplement. Any honey made through such a process is non-medicinal.

The majority of truly raw and natural honeys are found overseas. This is because honey is highly valued there, worth far more than Americans are accustomed to. Even directly from the villages certain honeys may cost exorbitant amounts, which would shock the average consumer. Here, beekeepers follow old-fashioned processes. One such group of honeys is bottled by Super-Market Remedies. This company has put my stamp of quality on the label. The honeys available include wild oregano, thistle, Canadian prairie, orange blossom, fir tree, and dandelion. All are 100% raw, that is uncooked. All are derived from bees which collect only natural food—no sugar is fed. Sugar-fed bees become diseased, and so does their honey. What's more, such honey is relatively inexpensive, the naturally fed bees produce less honey, which is highly valued. It is a health-booster not merely a food. For instance, the wild dandelion honey, which is exceedingly rare and which is derived from the Alpine mountain region, is some $25.00 per eight ounces. These honeys are difficult to find in stores. To order call 1-800-243-5242 or in Canada, 1-866-776-6550.

Papaya

This is the only fruit powerful enough to make the list of germ-killing foods. It is actually an enzyme within the fruit, specifically within the seeds, that is the killer. This enzyme, known as papain, not only kills directly but it also helps the white blood cells in their killing effort. This is because the white blood cells absorb the papaya enzyme, using it to digest microbes as well as cleanse or eradicate inflammation. The enzyme also improves blood flow, which prevents blood clotting. To stay in optimal health eat a papaya per week, but make sure it is organic, since this fruit is now genetically engineered. Also, eat the seeds. Mix the seeds in a blender with extra virgin olive oil, vinegar, oregano, and garlic; add a bit of the flesh for taste; as an additional taste sensation add a tablespoon or two of Pomegranate Syrup; blend and use as a peppery salad dressing.

Radishes

This hot vegetable is one of nature's finest medicines. In the United States it is a neglected food, relegated to a mere garnish.

Yet, it is readily available in all supermarkets. People should make extensive use of it for both the prevention of disease and to maintain a strong immunity.

Radishes contain sulfur compounds, which are significant antiseptics. Notice how long they remain in the refrigerator without molding. When they are eaten, this antiseptic is digested by the body and used to fight germs.

Radishes are one of nature's best sources of selenium, that is if they are grown in selenium-rich soil. In this case they act as a bona fide selenium supplement.

Well known for their tonic effects upon the gut radishes help stimulate the flow of critical digestive juices. In particular, they aid in bile secretion. This is a critical benefit. Bile is one of the body's main antiseptics. The regular flow of bile helps prevent internal infections.

Egg yolks

The yolk of raw eggs is a potent medicine. This is because egg yolks are super-rich in nutrients, which are direly needed by a weak body. Plus, eggs are rich in lecithin, a kind of germicide. The lecithin is an emulsifying agent, which means it mobilizes fat. This function is critical in severe viral infections. Viruses are coated with a fatty membrane. That membrane can be dissolved, which will destroy the virus. This is precisely what lecithin achieves. Lecithin is also found in soy, however, the type found in eggs is far more potent, especially against viruses. Eggs are also rich in vitamin B-6, which is needed for protein and antibody synthesis. Raw egg whites should not be consumed. They contain an enzyme which disturbs body chemistry.

While the whites are the main source of protein, egg yolks contain a considerable amount. The ingestion of raw protein is invaluable for the immune system, since protein is required for the building of all cells. The type of protein found in egg yolks is well tolerated by the body and is immediately absorbed. This protein is used in the building of healthy blood cells, including the germ-fighting white blood cells. It is also used to produce antibodies and interferon, crucial for the immune defenses.

The easiest way to eat raw egg yolk is to add it to a protein shake. Only organic eggs must be used. The Nutri-Sense makes an ideal medium for such a shake, because, while providing some protein it is a tasty and top source of natural vitamins. The combination of Nutri-Sense plus an egg yolk creates a super-nourishing drink that provides the cells with nutritional power. Here is the recipe for the most powerful and nutritious of all shakes:

- 1 or 2 egg yolks (from organic eggs only. To eliminate any risk of germs add a few drops of Oreganol P73)
- 3 tablespoons Nutri-Sense
- 1 cup full fat yogurt or 1 1/2 cup full fat milk
- handful pine nuts or blanched almonds
- 1 or 2 tablespoons raw honey (or for a natural chocolate-like taste, use Carob Molasses
- frozen berries
- water as needed
- extra lecithin (organic sunflower seed lecithin)

Note: this type of lecithin is only available via mail-order: 1-800-243-5242.

Blend thoroughly and drink as a super-nutritious meal. No other food is necessary. This maintains the appetite for several hours. This drink may be needed to help revive the body after a severe infection. It can also be taken as a daily tonic to increase overall resistance. Nutri-Sense provides rich amounts of niacin, pantothenic acid, natural vitamin E, and thiamine. The egg yolk provides excellent amounts of folic acid, riboflavin, niacin, pantothenic acid, lecithin, vitamin D, and vitamin E. The pine nuts provide protein and essential fatty acids, and almonds provide a vast array of nutrients, including vitamin E, amino acids, magnesium, calcium, phosphorus, riboflavin,

Yogurt

Humankind has always taken advantage of this blessed food. It is one of the most important preventive food/medicines known. Yogurt is medicinal, largely because of its bacterial content. It is the richest naturally occurring source of Lactobacillus acidophilus known.

Eli Metnikoff gave final proof for the powers of yogurt. He inoculated himself with a potentially fatal germ, cholera, drinking a bolus of water contaminated with this germ. Then, he drank a liter or more of yogurt, and never developed the disease. This demonstrates the immense value and power of natural foods in the prevention and treatment of disease. The body relies upon food and food-like substances for support, not chemicals.

Yogurt, taken regularly, is a major aid to immune health. It provides highly digestible proteins, which are readily used by the body. The proteins in yogurt are nearly 100% absorbed and are far more usable by the body than proteins from inferior sources such as beans, legumes (including soy), and grains. These proteins, which are constituted by the critical essential amino acids, are used by the body to produce the components of the immune system such as white blood cells and antibodies. Thus, yogurt provides the nutritional support needed for the maintenance of normal immunity.

Yet, yogurt's most invaluable contribution is its germs. A good grade of natural yogurt contains billions of them in the form of the healthy lactobacilli. These bacteria readily colonize the intestines, driving out noxious germs. There, they produce a wide range of valuable substances, including vitamins, enzymes, and antibiotics. Organic milk yogurt is significantly richer in key nutrients, as well as high quality acidophilus, than commercial types. What's more, commercial milk contains growth hormones, many of which are highly toxic. To gain the greatest benefits from yogurt therapy be sure to consume it regularly, like every day or every other day.

Certain individuals poorly tolerate milk products, even yogurt. In such individuals the consumption of yogurt might weaken the immune system. There is an alternative way to achieve yogurt's immune boosting benefits. Health-Bac is a natural healthy bacterial supplement, which strengthens immunity. The fact is it is more effective than yogurt in balancing the intestinal bacteria. This is perhaps the highest grade healthy bacterial supplement available, as is demonstrated by the following case history:

CASE HISTORY

Mr. K., a 45-year-old executive, was slated for a month-long trip in the Middle East. Here, he always succumbs to diarrheal illness, which wreaks havoc on his trip. This time he prepared his body by taking Health-Bac, a teaspoon in warm water twice daily. He continued to take the Health-Bac throughout his tour and also took the Oregacyn, taking them at opposing times. For the first time he was free of diarrhea and had a pleasant and rewarding trip, which he attributed to the Health-Bac. The fact is he had tried other brands of healthy bacteria previously, but they failed to work.

Spices: nature's antibiotics

Spices are among the most potent natural medicines known. Loaded with a wide range of minerals, vitamins, flavonoids, and aromatic oils, spices offer a natural chemistry unknown in the drug kingdom. The fact is recent studies show that certain spices are equally as powerful and in some instances more powerful than corresponding drugs. Spices have been determined to exhibit significant germ-killing properties. However, they are also exceptional antioxidants, far more powerful than mere vitamins and minerals. They are also nutrient dense, containing a considerable amount of minerals and to a lesser degree, vitamins. There is another category: flavonoids. Such compounds account for the finding that spices have antioxidant as well as antiinflammatory properties. What's mores, spices offer a kind of anesthetic action, which has also been attributed to the flavonoids.

Oregano

This common spice is a potent germ killer. Lab tests prove that it kills all types of germs, including bacteria, viruses, fungi, yeasts, molds, and parasites. No drug offers such a wide killing range. With the exception of anthrax every known germ has succumbed to it. Even anthrax was partially inhibited by it.

Oregano, that is the essential spice oil, readily kills viruses. Siddiqui, publishing in *Medical Science Research,* described complete disintegration of cold and flu viruses in a concentration less than 1%. He described its antiviral actions as "remarkable." Ijaz at Microbiotest Labs conducted an experiment against the human coronavirus, a category which causes both SARS and the common cold. Using the P73 spice oil blend, that is the Oreganol, viral levels were reduced from 5,000,000 per milliliter to about 100: all in a mere 20 minutes. Oregacyn, which is made from several wild spices, tested even better. It obliterated all traces of the virus in less than 20 minutes. Human studies indicate that, in fact, both Oreganol and Oregacyn kill viruses within the human body. In one instance the hepatitis C virus was destroyed directly within the body: right in the blood. The oil proved effective in killing over 99.9% of the viruses.

This raises the issue: what are the different uses of such supplements? Oreganol is the original wild oregano oil. It is a less aggressive version but still highly effective. The oil offers the benefit of being in a dropper bottle for easy administration, both internally and topically. A few drops under the tongue create a potent and immediate action. The under-the-tongue administration is the most physiological method. The region under the tongue, that is the sublingual region, has a direct blood supply. This means that the oregano oil gains immediate access to the blood. Plus, there is a direct connection between the sublingual region and the sinuses, where infection may be hidden. The oil is also invaluable because it can be applied topically. Here, the uses are numerous. These include applying to warts, cold sores, skin growths, moles, and shingles. It is also ideal for any itchy rash and/or hives.

For minor cases of eczema, such as the type in children, it proves invaluable. However, in severe cases of eczema and/or psoriasis topical application is ill advised. Rather, the ideal method is to take it internally or apply a 5% cream, that is the Oreganol cream. The oil is also effective for skin fungal infections, including ringworm, athlete's foot, and jock itch. It may be used vaginally, but only if it is diluted. Here, the Oreganol cream would be preferable. The oil is also ideal for children, as it is an effective rubbing agent on the chest. It may also be rubbed on the feet as often as needed. Here, it is highly effective, especially in infants or toddlers. A drop or two can be added to an infant's bottle (warning: be sure to use only an edible spice-based oil of oregano such as Oreganol P73, Vivitas, and Vitamin Shoppe).

The Oregacyn is a multiple-spice extract made exclusively from wild spices. Because of the synergy of these spices it is even more powerful than the oil. It is truly an adult capsule, although teenagers may also tolerate it. Oregacyn is unusually potent. As mentioned previously it destroyed all traces of the difficult-to-kill coronavirus, obliterating millions of these viruses in less than 20 minutes. The fact is this is an antiviral antibiotic, strictly from nature. Ideally, it is useful as a short course, when a person needs it. However, in the event of the possibility of sudden infections or epidemics it may be taken preventively: merely one capsule daily or every other day. Oregacyn is the ideal traveler's companion. It proves invaluable for preventing respiratory diseases, which, today, are a traveler's plague. A capsule or two a day also prevents another cause of dire misery: diarrhea. It is also useful in the treatment of this condition. Simply take one every hour until the diarrhea stops.

Yet, the ideal protocol is to use both, that is the oil under the tongue or in juice and the capsules. This will offer the most strategic protection against dire infectious diseases. For killer infections it will also make the difference between life and death. The fact is all other herbal medicines, for instance echinacea, goldenseal, and elderberry, are insignificant compared to the confirmed powers of wild oregano. It is wild oregano which must be relied upon to survive unmerciful infections. It is also the agent to depend upon to prevent such infections. Remember, the pandemic flu strikes quickly. What's more, it can kill quickly: before an individual even knows he/she is sick. There is no warning. Thus, prevention is the ideal approach. A typical preventive protocol is to take an Oregacyn once or twice daily along with five drops of the oil under the tongue twice daily.

Germ-a-Clenz, the emulsified spice oil spray, makes an invaluable addition to the protocol. This aromatic and pleasant spice oil spray cleanses dead air, while activating the senses. It also kills a wide range of germs. Use the Germ-a-Clenz as a throat spray whenever feeling a sensation of infection, irritation, or soreness. As a preventive, mist the household air daily. In particular, mist the air around but not directly over a baby's bed or in a sick room. Also, mist the fur of animals. Since it is completely safe it is ideal for use in the kitchen. In summary the ideal protocol is the use of the Oreganol 73 oil of wild oregano, the Oregacyn capsules, and the Germ-a-Clenz spray. This is the natural, in fact, divine, power that makes the difference between weakness and misery, perhaps death, and vital stamina. Regardless of the severity of the epidemic if the individual uses the triple-action protocol, he/she will survive. History proves it. During the 1918 flu pandemic in the United States there was a factory where no one died. It was a spice factory, which specialized in grinding cinnamon. Apparently, the fumes from the cinnamon, which the workers inhaled, as well as the dust, which permeated their clothes, protected them from both sickness and fatality. Spices work. They save lives. Take advantage of their powers: your life may depend upon it.

Cumin

This seed is one of the most ancient of all natural medicines. In the Mediterranean it grows wild. In ancient times it was harvested by Mediterranean peoples to be used both as food and medicine. Ancient records indicate that it found use for circulatory disorders, skin problems, and digestive disorders. Grieve in *A Modern Herbal* denotes a wide range of uses, even for poor skin tone and migraines.

Cumin stabilizes digestive function. It also boosts the function of the pancreas and liver, especially in relation to blood sugar metabolism. A Pakistani study documents that cumin has "insulin-like" functions. Cumin also boosts overall cellular defenses. It does so by increasing the synthesis of a key cellular enzyme system: glutathione peroxidase and glutathione-Stransferase. These enzymes are crucial for maintaining the health of cells through the elimination of toxins. The point is cumin helps maintain vital cellular function for all cells, including immune cells. The regular intake of cumin or cumin extracts (i.e. edible oil of cumin) helps keep the cells and organs vital and strong, increasing their resistance against infectious diseases. An oil of edible cumin is available. What's more, this spice is one of the active ingredients of the Oregacyn.

Allspice

Cornell University claims that allspice is a universal germicide. When tested against a wide range of bacteria, it killed them all. Allspice is a berry from a bush native to the Caribbean. Tests prove that it also kills mold and fungi.

Allspice can be purchased in any grocery store. Simply steep the dried berries in hot water. Drink with honey if desired as a regular beverage. An all-natural Oil of Allspice by North American Herb & Spice is available. Simply add a few drop to hot tea or in desserts or baked goods. A few drops mixed with honey is an ideal immune tonic for children as well as adults. Allspice has anti-pain properties, so the honey-oil of allspice mixture is ideal to soothe sore throats. Beware of commercial allspice oils which may be made from the leaves instead of the fruit.

Cinnamon

This is a potent germ killer. It is especially aggressive against molds and yeasts. This potent spice also possesses significant antibacterial properties. The cinnamon cure can be achieved through many forms. Powdered cinnamon is the weakest form, yet it is partially effective. Cinnamon sticks are more potent. They can be brewed into a fresh tea. Or, oil of edible cinnamon (in an olive oil base) may be used. The latter is highly aggressive; always take this oil with meals. This is a tasty way to reduce the risk of infection. Edible oil of cinnamon in an olive oil base made exclusively by North American Herb & Spice may be added to cold or hot cereal or as an additive to hot teas. Cinnamon is a potent antiviral agent and is a key component of Oregacyn. During a pandemic be sure to include cinnamon in the daily regimen or take an Oregacyn capsule daily.

Cinnamon is one of the active ingredients of a special supplement, which is specifically made for diabetics as well as hypoglycemics. Recent research confirms that this spice, as well as other pungent compounds such as cumin and myrtle, possesses significant blood sugar-regulating actions. Known as Oregulin, this has been shown in scientific studies to reduce the blood sugar by as much as 40%. The fact is because of its blood sugar controlling powers Oregulin is the ideal natural way to reverse this condition. What's more, preliminary studies show that regarding Syndrome X, that is the combination of high blood fats, high blood sugar, and high blood pressure, Oregulin is highly effective, both for high as well as low blood sugar. A mere capsule or two with meals is more effective than typical pharmaceutical drugs.

Cloves

As early as 1918 researchers discovered that cloves are germicidal. Using clove oil French investigators sterilized septic water. Recently, cloves have been touted as a parasite killer. Hulda Clark in her book *The Cure for All Cancers* claims that cloves are highly effective for killing a plethora of parasites, including intestinal and liver flukes. A study published by Cornell University documents how cloves kill a wide range of bacteria, including salmonella, shigella, staph, strep, and E. coli. In particular, clove oil contains substances which directly inhibit the growth of parasites, including flukes and worms.

The clove cure can be accomplished in a variety of ways. A number of bulk teas, such as those made by Republic of Tea, contain freshly dried cloves. Or, you can simply buy clove buds, which can be brewed into a tea. Edible oil of clove may also be consumed. Be sure that such an oil is from the edible clove bud rather than the inedible leaf. Or, for a potent and highly convenient dose take Oil of Clove Buds (North American Herb & Spice, 1-800-243-5242) one-half dropperful twice daily. This is the edible form of clove oil, which is different from the commercial oil. The edible type is made from the actual clove flower, i.e. the bud, while the commercial type is made from the inedible clove leaves and bark. Oil of edible Clove Buds is an ideal antiparasitic agent. Plus, it is invaluable for reversing digestive disorders as well as intestinal or stomach spasms.

Sage

A moderately powerful germicide, sage is one of the most ancient of all herbal medicines. The ancient proverb claims that if sage is readily used no disease will ever afflict the body. This is highly plausible. Sage not only kills germs but also dramatically strengthens the internal organs, especially the glands. It is one of the most potent antioxidants known. Plus, it is a highly effective hormonal tonic, balancing the function of the entire glandular system.

Sage is a primary component of Oregacyn antimicrobial formula. This herb is one of the most protective known for brain and nerve function. It has been used as a nerve tonic for thousands of years. It has been long known as an effective therapy for relaxing the nerves. It also has recently been shown to prevent memory loss and, in fact, regenerate nerve cell function. Recent studies indicate that wild sage, through its regenerative powers, boosts mental function and reverses memory loss, even in the aged. An exceptional form of wild sage is available as the active ingredient of Neuroloft. This is the wild sage from the Mediterranean mountains. This sage grows up to 8,000 feet above sea level. This is combined with wild rosemary and St. John's wort. For neurological imbalances take two or more capsules twice daily.

Recently, it was determined that sage is a potent agent for protecting the health of cells. It also possesses significant antiviral properties. What's more, it appears to strengthen the body against viral attack, that is it bolsters stamina. The regular intake of sage, a key component of Oregacyn, is a reliable way to avoid cold and flu attack.

Sage strengthens the adrenal glands. This may explain its power in warding off viral attack. The adrenal glands are greatly stressed by viral illnesses. By helping keep the adrenals strong and by boosting the immune response sage is an effective aid in the prevention of viral infections.

Antiseptic juices

Spicy vegetables are rich in oxygen. They also contain prodigious amounts of magnesium, which is needed for oxygen utilization. They are also rich sources of sulfur, which is a mild antiseptic.

Spicy vegetables contain a number of substances with germicidal actions. These substances include enzymes, including peroxidases, sulfur compounds, oxygenated compounds, hydrogen peroxide, and essential oils. Hot vegetables are more germicidal than bland ones. Consider radishes. Does anyone recall ever seeing them mold? In fact, this is rare. This is because the heat component in the radish is also a germ killer. When juicing, add a few drops of the Oreganol as a preservative, that is so none of the juice spoils. For more details regarding antiseptic juices see Recipes as Remedies (Chapter 6).

Antiseptic fruit

Certain fruits contain antiseptics. In general these are also the fruits which are rich in vitamin C. Citrus fruit contains the most powerful antiseptics. These are found largely in the rinds. To gain the benefit of these antiseptics it is important to eat the fresh fruit with as much of the inner peel as possible. This means that only organic fruit can be eaten, since the rind stores toxins such as pesticides and herbicides. Peel the organic fruit and retain the peel. Eat the inner lining, or scrape it out and add it to food. Grate the outer peel and add to hot tea or hot cider. Especially during the winter do not let citrus go to waste. Use all parts of it. Also, grate the outer coating and place in dishes. Set out throughout the house as aromatherapy. Or, add the grated powder to pump soaps and/or facial scrubs.

Chapter 5
Power Nutrients

Regarding epidemics it is the solutions that are important, not the hype. Incredibly, nature provides reliable answers. Yet, the synthetic world, the purely man-made methods, fail to provide such answers. This again demonstrates evidence for issues beyond the mundane. Lives are at risk, in fact, people are needlessly dying. Drugs which can cure emerging diseases are lacking. Yet, incredibly, simple foods, herbs, and spices are curative. Such a fact indicates that there truly is a purpose for life and that each human should do all that is possible to seek excellent health, physically, emotionally, mentally, and spiritually. Yet, the great bastion of power in terms of health is the physical. If the body is physically sound, virtually anything can be accomplished. If it is weak, little if anything can be achieved.

Nutrients are desperately needed by the body to keep it in optimal condition. Nutrients are derived from food. Thus, it is possible to gain a cure through common foods, which are rich in any missing factors. This is because a deficiency of even a single nutrient predisposes the body to disease, and this includes infectious conditions.

It is possible to find curative foods and various medicinal plants in the supermarket. Of course, health food stores are another source. So are farmer's markets. This is in regards to actual raw foods, in other words, many health food stores only carry supplements. So, health food markets and supermarkets, even farmer's markets, contain truly natural medicines. What's more, the vitamins and minerals from such foods are a kind of medicine. True, certain nutritional supplements offer such value, however, it is food and food-like substances which are the most potent as cures. Thus, natural-source vitamins and minerals are emphasized. The issue is if the individual gains as many of the needed vitamins and minerals from foods as possible, the results will be stupendous: vitality, strength, and heightened resistance.

The immune system rapidly burns up nutrients, especially if it is stressed. The fact is severe psychic stress can ultimately lead to immune collapse. A positive attitude greatly aids in immune health. Keeping upbeat, in fact, remaining as productive and spiritually high as possible—my dear friend Lamar Chapman calls it being spiritually productive—is the mainstay of strong immune health. What is spiritually productive? It is creating good will in yourself and among the people you encounter.

Yet, stresses do occur, and this results in the loss of key nutrients, notably vitamin C, vitamin A, zinc, and the B vitamins. A consistent effort must be made to replace any lost nutrients to keep the body in ideal health. A lack of certain key nutrients greatly predisposes the body to potentially rampant infections, including colds, flu, flesh-eating bacteria, tuberculosis, malaria, and hepatitis. The fact is microbes encounter great difficulty in establishing infection in the event of a powerful immune system.

The importance of vitamin A

This is one of the most crucial of all nutrients for strong immunity. A deficiency of this vitamin is relatively common.

This is largely because vitamin A-rich foods are relatively few. These foods include fatty fish, fish liver oils, seafood, such as lobster, crab, oysters, and mussels, butter, cream, whole milk, egg yolks, liver, and kidney. The failure to eat such foods leads to vitamin A deficiency. In fact, due to restrictive diets or various dietary concerns people are specifically avoiding vitamin A-rich foods. This is catastrophic. Such avoidance can lead to a severe vitamin A deficiency.

Nuts, legumes, grains, and beans, foods that millions subsist on, are devoid of this vitamin. This is why people in poor countries are vulnerable to infections, especially lung disorders. Vitamin A is needed to maintain the protective lining of the lungs. Without it, the lung tissues become sclerotic. Fruits and vegetables are also devoid of the vitamin. True, fruits and vegetables contain pro-vitamin A. However, there is no guarantee that this form will suffice the tissue needs. The issue is the body must be able to efficiently convert pro-vitamin A (i.e. beta carotene) to the biologically active form before this source may be regarded as significant. People who fail to properly convert beta carotene to useable vitamin A include diabetics, those with hypothyroidism, vegetarians, vegans, those with gallbladder disease, liver disorders, and people taking multiple medications. Regarding the latter it is the cholesterol-lowering drugs which are the primary culprits, as well as mineral oil. These drugs aggressively deplete this vitamin. In addition, people on a low fat diet are usually deficient in this vitamin, as well as its precursor, beta carotene. True, the latter is found in prodigious amounts in vegetation. Yet, its absorption is dependent upon dietary fat. A lack of fat in the diet leads to its malabsorption.

An adequate vitamin A status offers significant protection against disease. A lack of vitamin A weakens the body, greatly increasing the risks for infectious diseases, especially respiratory conditions. A low or deficient vitamin A content results in degeneration of lung tissues, particularly the critical cilia, which are largely responsible for preventing lung infection. To keep infections at bay it is crucial to maintain a regular intake of vitamin A-rich foods. This is a significant insurance against dangerous or killer infections.

Vegetarians get no vitamin A. Yet, this is an essential vitamin, a lack of which leads to a variety of symptoms, illnesses, and diseases. Common symptoms of vitamin A deficiency include night blindness, sensitivity of the eyes to bright light, dry skin, dry mucous membranes, dry eyes, increased vulnerability to infections, digestive disturbances, loss of the sense of smell, chronic sinus infections, and poor vision. Yet, there are dozens of other symptoms. For instance, a lack of vitamin A significantly increases the risks for yeast infections. For more information regarding vitamin A deficiency see the self-testing Web site, Nutritiontest.com. Here, the individual can define the exact level of his/her vitamin A deficiency. Advice on supplementation is included.

Vitamin D: the neglected player

Regarding immune health vitamin D is rarely mentioned. It is well known that vitamin D is the critical nutrient for bone health. It maintains bone density, which is critical not only for the skeleton but also for the immune system. The bones are the source of much of the immune power. This is because they house the immune cells' factories: the bone marrow. Here, at an incredible rate the white blood cells are synthesized. Billions of white blood cells are produced in its deep recesses daily. If the bones are weak, so is the bone marrow. Thus, the vitamin stimulates the development of strong bones and bone marrow. Diseases of the bones and bone marrow greatly disrupt immune function. Vitamin D helps keep these organ systems strong. Symptoms of vitamin D deficiency include joint pain, aching in the bones, aching in the teeth, chipping of the teeth, thinning of the bones, scoliosis, muscular spasms or rigidity, tooth decay, muscle twitching, and many others.

The regular intake of vitamin D results in considerable improvement of health, largely because of its effects upon the bone marrow. This vitamin greatly strengthens the tissues, especially the bones, joints, ligaments, and teeth, resulting in significant resistance against diseases. Societies where vitamin D intake is high are exceptionally healthy. What's more, the regular exposure to sunlight is also critical for improving health and resistance, largely because it boosts vitamin D levels. The vitamin then stimulates the deposition of both calcium and magnesium into bone. This may explain the observation that regular exposure to sunlight significantly improves bone density, since sunlight induces the synthesis of this vitamin-hormone. By increasing bone density and strengthening the health of the bone marrow vitamin D greatly aids immune health. It simply makes the individual stronger. What's more, it makes the skeleton strong, and ideal health is impossible without a strong skeletal structure.

Vitamin D is necessary for the absorption and utilization of calcium, magnesium, and phosphorus, all of which are critical for cellular health. Without it, the bones readily become depleted of these minerals. In other words, a lack of vitamin D leads to bone degeneration. Top sources of vitamin D include fatty fish, fish liver extracts, organic liver, sardines, fat-rich cheeses, whole milk, cottage cheese (full fat), kidney, and egg yolks. For many individuals on strict diets the majority of these foods are avoided. This is a nutritional catastrophe, since this vitamin is essential for overall health. For a more thorough evaluation of vitamin D status see the self-testing system, Nutritiontest.com.

It is critical to evaluate vitamin D status. In the event of a deficiency sudden breakdown of the body may readily occur.

This may result in spontaneous bone fractures, which may prove fatal. The fact is spontaneous fractures are common in individuals, particularly in strict vegans, who receive no dietary vitamin D. There is another dire consequence for vegans: a high phytic acid intake. The latter aggressively binds calcium, as well as magnesium, preventing its absorption. What's more, the vegan diet leads to stomach atrophy: if the stomach is never used for its purpose, that is the production of stomach acid for the digestion of animal foods, it atrophies. This leads to the inability to absorb calcium, since this mineral must be acidified to be absorbed. This explains why strict vegans frequently develop fractures, even from minor injuries. Why damage your body, that is when it is so brilliantly constructed? Avoid such damage by eating a variety of foods, including healthy animal products.

Avoid extremely strict diets, which do the body harm. Be moderate in dietary approach. If desiring a vegetation diet, add a few sources of animal foods such as organic yogurt or cheese or perhaps wild fish. If you follow a strict diet, which restricts or eliminates vitamin D-rich foods, be sure to take supplemental sources. The fact is a complete lack of vitamin D in the diet rapidly leads to bone loss, which may result in damage to the bones, joints, teeth, and even internal organs. One way to modify this is through herbal calcium sources. The OregaMax is a top source of a kind of wild calcium, phosphorus, and magnesium derived from mountainous rock. The wild oregano grows on the rock, concentrating these minerals. The fact is the trace minerals in OregaMax are among the most well absorbed and utilized known. Bone densitometry tests have shown that people who regularly take OregaMax, about six capsules daily, have the bone density of women half their age. Wild oregano is acidic, which aids in calcium absorption.

Case History:

Mrs. C. is a 40-year-old single mother, with a history of bone loss. Bone densitometry revealed a moderate case of osteoporosis. She began taking the OregaMax religiously, six or more capsules daily. After five months she had her results repeated: the bone density was normal, in fact, she had the bone mineral content of a 30-year-old. This was a dramatic improvement, all through the herbal source.

Vitamin C: Nature's immune chemical

While many people give accolades to vitamin C supplements as their protector, I have found that natural vitamin C, the kind found in fresh vegetables, fruit, herbs, and berries, is far superior to the synthetic type. The fact is synthetic vitamin C may contain residues of harmful chemicals, including solvents. Plus, it may be derived from genetically engineered corn. If this is the case, it is unfit for human consumption.

The regular intake of natural vitamin C offers significant protection against disease, including infections. Think about it. Natural vitamin C is a vital, living molecule. It is vitalized by the sun, and, thus, is full of solar energy. How could such a super-charged molecule be compared to laboratory manufacture? The laboratory molecule is sterile, devoid of vibrant energy. Upon testing it is molecularly dead, that is it fails to vibrate. The natural vitamin C, supercharged by the sun, vibrates, dances, and radiates with energy. That energy invigorates the body, giving it resistance against disease, providing it with the vitality it needs to ward off infection.

This vitamin C may be consumed both in food and supplements. However, only natural vitamin C supplements are vitalizing. Be sure the supplement you take is 100% natural in source. Labels are deceiving. You need proof from the company. Over 98% of all vitamin C supplements are synthetic. What's more, the vitamin C in these supplements is synthesized from corn sugars. The corn is largely genetically engineered. Avoid any such supplements. Instead, get your vitamin C from food as well as totally natural sources.

Purely-C is perhaps the only totally natural vitamin C supplement available. Made exclusively from natural sources it is an unprocessed herbal and food supplement. It is free of synthetic vitamins as well as genetically engineered contaminants. Purely-C contains a variety of novel sources of vitamin C and bioflavonoids, including red sour grape powder, wild strawberry leaves, Rhus coriaria, acerola cherry, rose hips, and camu camu berry. Regarding the latter it is perhaps the world's top source of vitamin C, containing 120 to 160 mg per gram. This variety of natural substances gives Purely-C great nutritional powers. It contains not only prodigious quantities of natural vitamin C but also rich amounts of naturally occurring bioflavonoids. The fact is it tastes like food. Thus, it is ideal to add to juices, shakes, or over salads/soups. What's more, it is acidic, which stimulates digestion. This is because it contains natural acids, which have tonic effects and which are entirely safe: tannic, malic, ascorbic, and gallic acids. Wild berries and herbs, such as camu camu berries, which originate from the Amazon forests, are the most potent and safe sources of this vitamin. Such substances are the active ingredients of Purely-C.

Pantothenic acid: power player

This vitamin keeps the body in a vital state. This is because pantothenic acid is involved in a life and death function: the output of the adrenal glands. The adrenal glands secrete steroids, which keep the internal organs fit. Without proper steroid secretion, the organ systems fail. Pantothenic acid is the key vitamin responsible for steroid synthesis. Without it the synthesis of these compounds declines and, ultimately, fails. The steroids are needed by every cell in the body. The deficiency greatly increases the vulnerability for infectious attack. The adrenal hormones, particularly cortisone, are needed for combating inflammation and tissue damage caused by stress and/or infection. The fact is cortisone is the body's anti-stress molecule. When cortisone levels decline, the body's resistance to stress, which includes the stress of infection, falters. Cortisone and, therefore, pantothenic acid, is a front line of defense against infection. Thus, it is critical to keep pantothenic acid intake high to resist or avoid pandemic diseases.

Vitamin B-6: immune protein builder

Throughout the body amino acid synthesis is dependent upon vitamin B-6. It is the most critical vitamin for the synthesis of antibodies, which are a type of immunological antibiotic. This vitamin is also needed for the creation of normal white and red blood cells.

Antibodies are critical for the immune defenses. These protein molecules are synthesized by the cells specifically for neutralizing bacteria. Without them, the immune system is direly weakened. Vitamin B-6 directly stimulates the production of these crucial immune proteins. A deficiency of this vitamin results in a dramatic decline in antibody synthesis. Top sources of vitamin B-6 are relatively rare and include tuna, fresh red meat, organ meats, poultry, and bananas. To determine personal B-6 nutritional status see the Web site, Nutritiontest.com.

Folic acid: total body tonic

Folic acid is critical for the maintenance of a strong immune system. This is because this vitamin is involved in virtually all aspects of organ, as well as immune, function. The synthesis of all cells, including the critical white blood cells, is dependent upon this vitamin.

Folic acid is the body's cellular sealant. It helps keep cells in a tight condition, which is important for the cells' resistance. In other words, it helps prevent the development of gaps between cells. This tightness of the cell membranes is the first line of defense against infection: tough, tight cell membranes are a powerful defense against germs. By keeping the germs from being able to invade, much of the battle is already won. Now, the germs founder, and the immune system is able to detect and destroy them, before they can enter the cells. Once germs break through the cell walls, they are able to hide, evading the immune response. Folic acid deficiency results in a weakening of the cellular cement. A lack of vitamin C also weakens this cement. This is why a deficiency of these vitamins leads to infections. When the deficiencies are extreme, the microbes are able to penetrate. Thus, the regular intake of folic acid, as well as vitamin C, in food and supplements significantly protects the body against infectious assaults.

Folic acid controls perhaps the most critical of all processes: the growth of cells. This includes the growth of immune cells. Thus, if this vitamin is lacking, the development of new white blood cells is sluggish. Plus, any existing cells are impaired in function.

Folic acid is readily destroyed. Solvents, chemicals, food additives, and excessive heat all inactivate it. Perhaps the most vile offender is alcohol, which is an effective antagonist. A mere drink a day is enough to destroy within a week or two virtually all folic acid within the tissues.

There are dozens of symptoms of folic acid deficiency. The primary symptoms include hang nails, lips which are constantly chapped, muscle or leg cramps, digestive disturbances, colitis.

diarrhea, receding gums, persistent infections, poor wound healing, fatigue, and poor circulation. The best food sources of this nutrient include fresh organic red meat, poultry, organic liver, eggs, rice bran, rice germ, spinach, parsley, almonds, broccoli, and cauliflower. To determine your folic acid needs you may test yourself for the deficiency. To do so see the Web site, Nutritiontest.com, or call 1-800-243-5242. Through the nutritiontest system the individual can determine his/her exact folic acid status, plus corrective recommendations. The same is available through the book *Nutrition Tests for Better Health* (Dr. Cass Ingram, 2004).

Zinc: immune regulating mineral

A critical aid to natural resistance zinc controls a wide range of immune functions. The health of the thymus, lymph glands, liver, spleen, and bone marrow are all dependent upon it. Blood cell activity is highly dependent upon this mineral. What's more, the synthesis of key hormones, such as thymic hormone and insulin, are zinc dependent. Many of these hormones, notably thymic and thyroid hormones, exert antibiotic-like action.

Zinc itself is a mild antiseptic. In the 1800s zinc chloride was used post-surgically to prevent wound infections. A solution of zinc chloride of sulphate completely destroys virtually any germ. During the 1800s doctors claimed that applications of zinc chloride post-surgically prevented infections, while causing a dramatic healing of wounds. Zinc is required for protein synthesis, that is the incorporation of amino acids into the cell. The rebuilding of all cell components is zinc-dependent. So is the repair and rebuilding of genetic material.

Without this mineral the immune system becomes dysfunctional. Thus, in order to keep this system in optimal condition proper zinc nutrition must be adhered to. Zinc is found in relatively few foods, with red meat being the top source. Other excellent sources include fish, crab, oysters, lobster, poultry, eggs, peanuts, peanut butter, and pumpkin seeds. Whole grains are a relatively poor source, since they contain zinc antagonists known as phytates. Wild oregano is also an excellent source. OregaMax provides micro-amounts of natural zinc, a kind of "homeopathic" dosing, which helps reestablish zinc stores. The micro-doses are invaluable and greatly aid in improving cellular nutrition. The type of zinc in OregaMax is completely bioavailable. Chelated zinc supplements may prove invaluable, that is in building up zinc stores and replacing any lost zinc. The fact is this mineral is readily lost through the urine and stool. What's more, deficiency is common and is manifested by a wide range of symptoms, including fatigue, muscle weakness, joint pain, skin disorders, including dry or rough skin, hair loss, white spots on the nails, increased vulnerability to infections, lack of appetite, loss of the sense of taste, infertility, impotence, swollen prostate, lack of the sense of smell, poor wound healing, blood sugar disturbances, and repeated skin infections (including acne).

People who eliminate red meat from the diet routinely become zinc deficient. This is because in the American diet red meat is the top food source. Turkey is an acceptable alternative, since it is nearly as rich as beef and lamb in this mineral.

Selenium: cellular guardian

Selenium may be regarded as the anti-toxin mineral. This is because it helps the cells form a defense against damage by virtually any toxin or germ. Selenium forms a critical part of a potent defense system known as glutathione peroxidase. This is the cells' front line of defense against toxic invasion, particularly exposure to noxious chemicals, poisons, and toxic injuries. The enzyme glutathione peroxidase, which is bound to four selenium atoms, intercepts toxins before they damage cells.

Selenium deficiency greatly impairs immunity. It increases the risks for both cancer and heart disease. This is because in the event of its deficiency the synthesis of glutathione fails.

Selenium may be difficult to procure in the diet. Levels in food are dependent upon where the food is grown. Some soils are naturally high in selenium, while others are low. States with high or acceptable selenium levels include South Dakota, Texas, and some parts of California. States with very low levels include Illinois, Michigan, Indiana, Ohio, western New York, Massachusetts, Vermont, Rhode Island, Connecticut, Maine, Oregon, and Washington. Note that many of these states are in the Great Lakes region. The soil of this region was extensively depleted during the glacier age, when these massive structures ground away untold billions of tons of fertile topsoil, rich in selenium, from the region. Coastal regions are also depleted, the selenium being washed from the shore through erosion.

Symptoms of selenium deficiency are often vague. However, heart disorders, especially enlarged heart, weakened heart, and cardiomyopathy, are cardinal. Other symptoms of the deficiency include weak immune system, allergic tendencies, premature aging of the skin, brown spots, and infertility. For a more thorough evaluation of the deficiency see the Web site, Nutritiontest.com

Healthy cell membranes: key to protection

The body has a number of mechanical barriers for preventing infection. These barriers include the skin, digestive linings, and, on a microscopic level, cell and nuclear membranes. Such barriers are the front line of defense against infection. Cell membranes, if healthy, are a significant barrier against the entry of germs into the cells. These membranes are highly selective regarding what they allow to enter. Thus, they permit the entry of nutrients, while obstructing the entry of germs. However, if the membranes are damaged or diseased, then the germs may enter more readily. If they are weak, they are more readily attacked by the germs, resulting in the invader's entry. The nuclear membrane is also highly selective; germs have a difficult time penetrating it.

Viruses fail to infect the body, as long as they are unable to attach to cell walls. Again this virus-cell wall interaction is critical, because this is the first barrier of defense. Thus, if the appropriate defenses are available, infection can largely be prevented. There are ways to strengthen the cell wall defenses. Viruses begin infections by fusing with the cell wall, and this is particularly true with the so-called fatty membrane-coated viruses. If this fatty coating can be disrupted, the virus fails to attach. This demonstrates the role of natural solvents in disabling or destroying viruses. Plus, if the cells' coating is exceptionally strong, the virus has a difficult time attaching. Cells which are damaged or aged can become stiff, that is the membranes become taut or brittle. These damaged and/or aged membranes are more readily attacked by viruses, which explains the high vulnerability of the elderly to such infections. It is well known that the elderly suffer from cellular breakdown, and this includes the cell membranes. That aged appearance seen externally is also occurring on the cellular level. How can a person keep their membranes fluid? It is through solid nutritional practices and through the ingestion of special foods known as fluid membrane enhancers. The fatty compound known as lecithin is perhaps the most important of these. Found in a wide range of foods, the best sources are organ meats, whole soy beans or whole soy bean foods, whole milk products, full fat cheese, butter, and eggs. The latter are a top source of these membrane enhancers. This is because eggs, that is egg yolks, are a dense source of a special kind of lecithin, which is rapidly absorbed. The cell membranes thrive on this type of lecithin, which helps make them more fluid. Lecithin is also found in nuts and nut butters, however, the ideal type is found in animal foods. Milk products are another excellent source of animal lecithin. These sources include whole organic milk, organic full fat cottage cheese, and imported or raw cheeses. Butter contains a significant amount of lecithin. If you are allergic to it, look for goat butter. The regular intake of such foods dramatically increases the flexibility of cell walls, increasing their resistance against viral attack. However, be sure to eat only organic sources. Vegetarians may procure significant amounts of lecithin from avocados, soy, nuts, seeds, and nut butters. However, such foods are lacking in cholesterol, which works in concert with the lecithin. Without cholesterol the synthesis of a wide range of critical substances falters. Cell walls become diseased. As a result, germs may readily attack and invade them. The fact is cholesterol is a key defense for cells against germ invasion.

There are two key components to resistant cell membranes: flexibility and strength. The basis of this is the cell wall proteins and fatty acids. These substances are derived directly from the diet. Thus, if the diet consists of healthy and uncorrupted sources of these foodstuffs, this will be directly represented within the cell walls. This is the basis for the statement that people are what they eat. If the proteins are excessively heated or incomplete, the cell walls will suffer. If the fatty acids are excessively processed or adulterated, this will directly impact cellular health. The cell wall must be strong for the body to fight and resist disease. Thus, care must be taken regarding the kinds of fats, oils, and proteins which are consumed as well as how such foods are processed and/or cooked. Oils and fats especially should be eaten in the raw or minimally processed state. Oils which are aggressively heated will cause cell damage. Top quality oils which help maintain cell wall flexibility include raw organic butter, raw organic egg yolk (or gently cooked yolk), cold pressed nut oils, raw nuts (or lightly cooked nuts), and raw (or lightly cooked) seeds. Excellent sources of protein include raw nuts and seeds, raw or mildly heated egg yolks, raw milk, raw milk cheese, raw milk yogurt, and rare meat. Regarding the latter only beef and lamb from organic sources can be eaten rare. When eating such meat, be sure to take as a protective a few drops of Oreganol. Heat fails to destroy prions. So, cooking temperature may fail to be protective. Yet, gain as much benefit from the oil as possible; rub all steaks, chops, and roasts with a thin layer of it.

Cholesterol: the unsung hero

Cholesterol is a potent defender against infection. It has been unfairly maligned. The fact is this substance is required for the health of all cells. Without it the body degenerates. Critical organs, such as the brain, adrenal glands, ovaries, liver, gallbladder, and testes, which are dependent upon cholesterol, decay. For instance, various liver diseases, including hepatitis, cirrhosis, liver infection, and gallstones, may be directly caused by a low cholesterol diet. So can diseases of the brain, since this organ is highly dependent upon this substance. The brain cells thrive on a cholesterol-rich diet, while quickly degenerating if this substance is removed from the diet. The fact is a high cholesterol diet is one of the most reliable assurances against brain or nerve tissue infection. Thus, individuals who suffer from various neurological conditions may greatly benefit from a high cholesterol diet, since this substance emulsifies fat, preventing gallstone formation. Cholesterol is necessary for the synthesis of bile, which is the body's fat emulsifying agent. Without cholesterol, the liver and gallbladder become stagnant, leading to liver congestion, liver cell damage, and, of course, gallstones. The fact is the low fat diet is a primary cause of gallstone formation. One way to prevent gallstones is to regularly consume heavy oils, particularly extra virgin olive oil. This oil aids in bile production, keeping the liver secretions flowing.

Cholesterol is also needed by the immune system. All white blood cells require considerable amounts to remain healthy. Cholesterol is a critical component of the white blood cell membrane, greatly strengthening it, while keeping it fluid. Without this molecule, the cell membranes stiffen, reducing their ability to destroy bacteria. A highly fluid membrane causes the white blood cells to move in a more optimal fashion, so they can seek, trap, and kill invaders. Thus, it is crucial for the individual to eat plenty of cholesterol-rich foods in order to ensure optimal white blood cell health.

Boosting cellular energy reserves: another key defense

Cells require energy. If their energy reserves are low or depleted, they are greatly weakened. Weakened cells bode trouble, because they become highly vulnerable to disease and infection. This can be prevented by maintaining optimal cellular energy stores. The main source of energy for the cells is a phosphorus compound known as ATP. This substance provides explosive energy power for the cells; note that phosphorus is the substance which is used to make powerful bombs. So, ATP is the cells' power molecule, without which its function ceases.

ATP levels within the cells can be readily boosted. The fact is according to Arnold Levine, in his book, *Viruses*, cells have perfected the 'technology' to produce tremendous amounts of this molecule. He describes how, incredibly, a single liver cell can produce tens of millions of molecules of ATP every second. Considering the uncountable billions of cells within the body the amounts of ATP produced are incomprehensible. Thus, any defect in the production of this molecule increases the vulnerability to disease. Viruses rob the genetic machinery of its ATP production. They rob this production for themselves. This is why viral infections cause such dire fatigue. The cells are robbed of their energy source and, thus, there is no fuel to operate the body. For energy production to be normalized the virus must be killed.

ATP is made in a specialized intracellular factory known as the mitochondria. This miraculous structure is a kind of cell within the cell. It is a living entity, required for human existence. The mitochondria is a kind of living factory, where energy is produced from food. Its primary raw material is glucose, which is derived from various foods. The mitochondria is supported by a special membrane, which houses a spectacular array of amino acids, enzymes, vitamins, and minerals, all of which are used to synthesize energy. Again, each mitochondria makes millions of energy molecules every day, and there are trillions of these in the human body. Once these energy molecules are produced, they are released into the cell fluids to be used in the various cellular reactions. The mitochondria require certain substances for optimal operation. By supplying these organelles with what they need, energy production can be maximized. The body is a dependable structure. If it is provided with what it needs, it will adapt: it will empower itself, taking advantage of any support it is given. Thus, by manipulating the nutritional intake, the cellular energy production can be dramatically boosted, which provides one of the most potent defenses against dangerous diseases.

Again, ATP is made from the processing, that is the combustion, of glucose. Raw honey is an ideal source of this molecule. The kind of sugars in raw honey are readily absorbed and well tolerated by the body. This is why it is the ideal food during severe viral infections. It supplies the necessary fuel, so that the cells can build up energy stores for fighting off the invader. Other nutrients needed for the creation of energy include amino acids, riboflavin, niacin, vitamin C, phosphorus, and magnesium. Other foods/substances which boost ATP levels include wild oregano herb, i. e. the OregaMax, which is the whole unprocessed herb in a maximum dose, organically raised meats, whole milk products, egg yolks, nuts, seeds, and nut/seed butters.

Chapter 6
Recipes as Remedies

Now more than ever before it is important to know home remedies. The entire population must know the medicinal use of foods as well as food-like extracts. The following provides recipes and formulas on how to use the most potent medicinal foods to both stay well and get well.

Food has specific medicinal properties. For instance, blueberries contain flavonoids, which are invaluable for visual disorders. Cranberries contain an acid which helps reverse kidney troubles and bladder disorders. Onions contain a compound which thins the blood. Eggs contain a substance which helps reverse anemia, while fatty fish contains a compound which reduces inflammation. The fact is food is the ideal medicine. This is because it is both safe and effective.

How to use food as medicine

It is critical to know how to use food, that is as a cure. The germs are striking so fast and so unpredictably that modern medicine is incapable of responding. Thus, is there any other option other than self-care? There will come times when no other option will be available. Natural medicines cure without risk for serious side effects. Thus, they are the ideal therapies for use during crises. In the event of global disasters are there any other options? As cures drugs are impotent, in fact, dangerous. People must have a prescription to use them. No prescription is necessary for natural juices, extracts, honey, herbs, or spices. All these substances possess curative properties. Some are outright cures, even for life-threatening conditions. Now you will learn how to use these natural medicines, both for everyday needs and medical crises. There is much research to prove their efficacy. Plus, personal experience proves they work. Trust in the powers of nature. Let nature be the cure. It is reliable: there is no doubt about it.

Antiseptic juices

Antiseptic juices save lives. I have used them in my practice repeatedly with phenomenal success. These juices contain the full compliment of nutrients, all in the proper ratio. Thus, they provide optimal nourishment to the tissues. Plus, they contain potent plant chemicals capable of killing germs.

There is no question that plants possess germ-killing properties. This has been fully proven in scientific research. Put simply, antiseptic juices are effective, and the result is noticed quickly.

A wide range of plants contain germicides. Some of these germicides are weak and others exceptionally potent. Many, for instance, the juice of yellow onions or fresh garlic, are capable of killing virtually every germ known. Others not only kill but also provide additional actions, invaluable for infectious diseases. Ginger is an excellent example. The juice of fresh ginger kills the majority of germs. Yet, unlike garlic juice it soothes the stomach and halts both stomach and intestinal cramps. In contrast, while garlic kills most germs it causes gastric upset: even gastric ulceration.

Note: The power of each juice is rated either mild, moderate, or extreme.

Radish-Onion Juice (Extreme)

1 to 2 bunches red radishes, thoroughly washed
4 medium yellow onions
1 or more bunch parsley

Make a juice of these ingredients to taste. Add a few drops of the Oreganol, as a tonic and preservative. Vary the quantities of vegetables to taste. Drink as needed.

Spicy Greens Juice

This juice is high in antiseptic sulfur compounds as well as vitamin C. Watercress provides a rich amount of calcium. Arugula provides a mild antiseptic, which is effective within the liver and intestines. The fact is this juice essentially reverses intestinal disorders. Both watercress and arugula stimulate the function of the spleen, a critical immune organ. Parsley is a mild urinary antiseptic and diuretic, plus it is rich in folic acid, vitamin C, and magnesium.

fresh organic mustard greens
fresh organic watercress
fresh organic arugula
fresh organic parsley
fresh organic ginger

Make a juice of these ingredients in any amount/combination to taste. Add a few drops of the Oreganol, as a tonic and preservative. Drink as needed.

Purple Vegi Juice (moderate)

This juice is high in purple flavonoids, which exert significant antiseptic actions. Onions provide germicides helpful within the intestines, liver, kidneys, spleen, and blood. Cabbage contains mild antiseptics helpful within the intestines and stomach. Beets provide an antiseptic, betaine, mildly active within the liver and intestines.

    4 medium-size purple onions
    1 head purple cabbage
    1 or 3 raw beets (include well washed greens, if possible)

Make a juice of these ingredients to taste. Add a few drops of the Oreganol, as a tonic and preservative. Drink as needed.

Gingerized Carrot-Beet Juice

Beets have a mild antiseptic action, mainly on the liver and intestines. Carrots are added due to their rich beta carotene content, needed to make the mildly antiseptic vitamin A. The vitamin A can only be properly made if a person's thyroid is functioning optimally.

    organic ginger root
    organic carrots
    organic beets

Make a juice of equal proportions carrot and beet; add ginger until noticeable hot taste is achieved.

Protective meals

The following menus are based on high protein and high vitamins A and D. This is in order to create the strongest immune system possible. This is the type of menu which was lacking during the 1918 flu pandemic. Then, nutrition was notoriously poor. People were in a weakened state. The average person ate mostly carbohydrates, largely from bread. The epidemic could spread easily, and because people lacked resistance, they readily died. The diet is also high in vitamin C, vitamin B-6, pantothenic acid, selenium, and zinc, all of which potentiate the immune system. Vitamins B-6 and pantothenic acid are greatly needed for stimulating antibody synthesis. Vitamin C is needed for all immune functions and is quickly destroyed by stress, infection, or fever. Zinc and selenium are critical both for white blood cell function and antibody synthesis.

When the immune system is challenged, if it is lacking in key nutrients, it is unable to respond sufficiently. Thus, it is crucial to keep it well nourished. Such nourishment is achieved by a comprehensive dietary plan. The diet must be rich in nutrient-dense foods, that is foods which have a high amount of nutrients per calorie. In contrast, foods which have a high amount of calories but are low in nutrients should be avoided. The latter may be called "nutrient-poor" foods. Such foods include white flour, white bread, pasta (i.e. that made from white flour), corn products, white rice, candy, cookies, pies, doughnuts, cakes, ice cream, and similar foods. These foods greatly deplete immune power, not only because they are often contaminated with chemicals and additives but also because they simply lack the nutrients needed for strong immunity. Examples of nutrient-dense foods include whole unprocessed organic meats, including beef, lamb, poultry, and fish, as well as nuts and seeds, whole milk products, eggs, fresh fruit, and fresh vegetables. Fresh frozen vegetables are also nutrient dense. Corn is the exception. It is relatively low in nutrients. In general, the consumption of corn weakens the immune system. This is largely because commercial corn is high in mold residues, often containing the highly toxic aflatoxin. What's more, corn is relatively low in the immune-boosting amino acid, lysine. Beans are also relatively low in critical amino acids, as well as vitamins and minerals, since they are mostly carbohydrate. Thus, the latter have a high amount of calories per nutrient. The following is a list of the foods containing the highest nutrient density in order of most to least dense:

beef
lamb
duck
chicken
fish
eggs
seafood
whole milk products
seeds
nuts
the brans of grains
legumes, i. e. soy, lentils, beans
grains
baked and sweet potatoes
vegetables
fruit
raw honey

This is an impressive list. The majority of people have switched from such a diet, emphasizing foods which are rich in sugars and starches such as bread, pasta, potatoes, and fruits, all of which are relatively low in nutrients. From a point of view of immune strength this is disastrous. This is because nutrient density is the key to strengthening the immune system. This does not mean that an individual must live exclusively on animal foods. Nor should the individual presume commercial meat products and milk as safe. The commercial meat/milk industry is significantly compromised regarding safety. What's more, farmers are victims, that is of an agricultural and industrial monopoly, which controls the availability of options. The reason animal foods are included is that the regular intake of animal foods provides a high amount of the nutrients needed for healthy immunity. These include nutrients which cannot be procured from any other source. The fact is, ideally, such animal foods should be supplemented with high quality whole grains, nuts, potatoes, fruit, etc.

What's more, there are lists within the lists. For instance, fruit may be ranked in nutrient density. The following is a list of the most nutrient dense fruit, from most to least:

avocado

olives

strawberries

papaya

cantaloupe

tomato

kiwi

blueberries

grapefruit

orange

lemon/lime

Vegetables may also be ranked. Few vegetables are truly nutrient-dense. The following is a list of the most nutrient dense vegetables:

broccoli
spinach
parsley
cauliflower
Brussels sprouts
cabbage
cauliflower
watercress
red sweet pepper

Protein sources may also be ranked. For instance, fish and seafood vary in nutrient density, as follows:

salmon
sardines
herring
tuna (albacore)
tuna (yellow fin)
halibut
trout (fresh water)
crab
lobster
shrimp
oysters

Note the difference in the tuna. Albacore tuna lives in colder water and, therefore, is a richer source of the highly nourishing fatty fish oils than regular, that is yellow fin tuna.

Even oils may be ranked. For many the results may be surprising:

butter
crude pumpkinseed oil
extra virgin olive oil
avocado oil
crude rice bran oil
crude hazelnut oil
crude almond oil
sesame seed oil (unrefined)
sunflower seed oil (crude cold-pressed)
flaxseed oil

Butter is selected first, because of its high density of fuel fats needed for cellular metabolism. Incredibly, in particular the heart relies extensively on fuel fats, preferring the highly dense or saturated fats found in butter and heavy vegetable oils, like extra virgin olive oil and avocado oil. Extra virgin olive oil is the ideal alternative for those who are allergic to butter. It may be mixed with coconut fat to make a spread. Note that oils high in polyunsaturates, such as flaxseed and sunflower seed oil, are low on the list. The cells prefer heavy fats, such as monounsaturated oils, as fuel sources, and, thus, high polyunsaturated oils are less desirable. However, they do have a critical component: the essential fatty acids. Thus, it is critical to include a small amount of them in the diet, like a tablespoon daily.

Currently, there is a craze to consume flaxseed oil. Yet, incredibly, from a nutrient density point of view it would be superior to consume crude extra virgin olive oil, butter, or crude pumpkinseed oil that is the Pumpkinol, as a daily tonic than flaxseed oil. The flaxseed oil could be used as an occasional supplement, strictly as a source of essential fatty acids. Yet, crude cold-pressed pumpkinseed oil provides the essential fatty acids in an equally bioavailable form, plus it contains a higher degree of nutrient density, since it is exceptionally rich in vitamin E, provitamin A, and chlorophyll. Plus, it is far more digestible and is unlikely to cause intestinal, gastric, and skin irritation, a common consequence of flaxseed oil. The fact is unprocessed pumpkinseed oil fortified with essential oils (i.e. Pumpkinol) is perhaps the most digestible of all seed oils. It is the ideal vegetable oil for those who fail to tolerate olive oil. Pumpkinseed oil is derived from a common nutrient dense food; flaxseed oil is derived from a plant of minimal nutritional value.

These lists explain the rationale for the diet in the forthcoming section. It is a diet based exclusively upon nutrient density, not on any specific moral or philosophical basis. There is no attempt herein to impose a type of "meat-ism." Rather, it is strictly an issue of nutrient sufficiency, that is gaining the greatest amount of nutrients--amino acids, fatty acids, vitamins, minerals, enzymes, and flavonoids, per calorie, in fact, per ounce. Recipes which call for ingredients from commercial sources, which may not be safe, for instance, strawberries (due to pesticide contamination), milk (due to bovine growth hormone), or meat (due to commercial farming practices) imply organic sources only.

TWO WEEK MENU

Day 1

Breakfast
- Grass-fed beefsteak plus organic eggs (2 eggs over easy: this keeps the vitamin A intact)
- Large glass grapefruit juice (fresh squeezed is best; contains vitamin C, folic acid, and potassium)
- Slices of red sweet peppers (source of vitamin C)

Lunch
- Sardine salad (place the contents of one or two cans of sardines over a large bed of mixed salad greens; drizzle with extra virgin olive oil and vinegar)
- mineral water or V-8 juice

Supper
- Roast organic chicken with skin (skin is high in vitamins A, D)
- steamed broccoli (drink any remaining juice; high in vitamin C and potassium)
- Baked sweet potato (high in pro-vitamin A and vitamin E)

Day 2

Breakfast
- Bowl full fat organic cottage cheese dusted with tablespoon of Nutri-Sense (provides vitamins A and D and protein, plus B vitamins); top with fresh fruit, i.e. papaya, kiwi, and/or strawberries
- One or two pieces of whole grain or sprouted grain bread (coarse type found in health food stores); use crude raw honey as a spread

Lunch
- Ground organic hamburger mixed with chopped onions and garlic (provides amino acids for making blood cells and immunoglobulins; also provides germ-killing sulfur compounds)
- Salad of tossed mixed dark greens; top with extra virgin olive oil and vinegar

Supper
- Baked wild salmon or halibut (provides immune-building protein and fatty acids; the fatty acids are antiinflammatory); bake with slices of red onions and ginger
- Tossed green salad with chopped turnips and radishes; don't be skimpy on the latter. Add at least a half turnip and several radishes. Drizzle with extra virgin olive oil and vinegar
- Bowl organic strawberries in heavy cream or whole milk

Day 3

Breakfast
- Mediterranean egg omelet using three organic eggs cooked in extra virgin olive oil with diced green onions, feta cheese, and diced red pepper
- Glass fresh-squeezed orange juice
- Bowl oat bran cereal topped with raw honey, real whole organic milk (or cream) Note: cream or whole milk provides vitamins A and D as well as riboflavin, needed to oxygenate the tissues.

Lunch
- Wild salmon on a bed of mixed greens. Drizzle with extra virgin olive oil and fresh lemon juice
- Baked squash or sweet potato
- Mixed green salad with plenty of cherry tomatoes

Supper
- Baked wild salmon or halibut (provides immune-building protein and fatty acids; the fatty acids are antiinflammatory); bake with slices of red onions and ginger (Note: take a dropperful of the GreensFlush to detoxify the mercury)
- Tossed green salad with chopped turnips and radishes; don't skimp on the latter; add at least a half turnip and several radishes; drizzle with extra virgin olive oil and vinegar
- Bowl blueberries or blackberries in heavy cream or whole milk

Day 4

Breakfast
- Nutri-Sense shake made with whole fat yogurt, three tablespoons Nutri-Sense, frozen blueberries, and raw honey
- Large glass fresh-squeezed grapefruit juice
- Boiled egg

Lunch
- Strip steak or similar 8 oz steak (grass fed or organic)
- Baked potato with real butter and sour cream
- Bowl strawberries; to drizzle with raw honey

Supper
- Baked free range chicken (provides immune-building protein and fatty acids)
- Tossed green salad with chopped turnips and radishes; don't be skimpy on the latter; add at least a half turnip and several radishes; drizzle with extra virgin olive oil and vinegar
- Melon or sliced kiwi fruit

Day 5

Breakfast
- Ground organic turkey patty or turkey sausage. Eat with mustard
- Bowl oat bran cereal topped with crude raw honey and real cream or whole milk
- Glass fresh-squeezed orange or tangerine juice

Lunch
- Chopped radish, turnip, and parsnip salad; blend in crude pumpkinseed oil (Pumpkinol) and balsamic vinegar. Add a few cherry tomatoes for vitamin C. Also, add grapefruit sections
- Pomegranate Surprise (add 2 tablespoons Pomegranate Syrup to a glass sparkling water with or without ice)
- Large ground beef patty; top with cheese and eat with mustard and unsweetened ketchup (i.e. Westbrae's Unketchup)

Supper
- Roast leg of lamb (organic-grass fed)
- Hot greens and lettuce salad using mustard greens, watercress, arugula, and romaine lettuce
- Mixed fruit cocktail
- Herbal tea with raw oregano honey

Day 6

Breakfast
- Nutri-Sense shake
- 1/2 grapefruit
- 1 boiled egg
- Hot herbal tea

Lunch
- Organic strip steak of any kind
- Baked potato or fried potatoes (in extra virgin olive oil)
- Bowl strawberries or mixed berries; top with heavy cream, if desired

Supper
- Lamb chops (organic/grass fed) cooked medium-rare in lemon-garlic-oregano sauce
- Baked squash or sweet potato
- Mixed greens salad with plenty of sliced radishes and turnips
- Pomegranate Surprise

Day 7

Breakfast
- Bowl brown rice cereal; top with Nutri-Sense and whole milk; add crude raw honey for taste
- 2 poached eggs
- Glass fresh-squeezed grapefruit juice

Lunch
- 2 cans sardines in mustard sauce
- glass tomato juice
- mixed raw vegetables

Supper
- Roast beef drizzled with Pomegranate Syrup
- Home-made mashed potatoes (or baked potato)
- Spinach in lemon sauce
- Blueberries with cream and raw honey

Day 8

Breakfast
- Naturally raised elk, turkey, or chicken sausages
- Bowl oat bran cereal
- Pomegranate Surprise (2 tablespoons Pomegranate Syrup in spring or sparkling water on ice)

Lunch
- Huge mixed greens salad topped with organic full-fat cottage cheese and raw sunflower or pumpkin seeds; drizzle with extra virgin olive oil and vinegar.
- Mixed diced melon
- Glass mineral water

Supper
- Organic lamb chops in lemon-olive oil sauce
- Pomegranate Surprise or grapefruit juice (aids in the digestion of meat)
- Brussels sprouts in butter or extra virgin olive oil
- Baked sweet potato (drizzle with crude pumpkinseed oil)

Day 9

Breakfast
- Miscellaneous nut butters on cheese and vegetables; dust with Nutri-Sense
- Glass V-8 juice

Lunch
- Lemon or lime water
- Home-made hash containing chopped potatoes, beef, and onions

- Chopped variety root salad, containing parsnips, parsley root, green onions, turnips, and radishes

Supper
- Roast organic chicken pieces (leave skin on)
- Steamed broccoli or cauliflower (both are high in naturally occurring vitamin C; if there is any juice remaining in the cooking fluids, drink it)
- Baked potato (be sure to eat the skin, since it is rich in vitamin C and selenium)

Day 10

Breakfast
- Bowl full-fat organic cottage cheese (top with Nutri-Sense and diced melon of your choice)
- Glass grapefruit juice
- 1 to 2 boiled eggs

Lunch
- Fresh wild fish of any kind; squeeze a full lemon over it (note: lemon helps detoxify heavy metals, such as mercury, which is a contaminant in most fish)
- Steamed broccoli or Brussels sprouts
- Tea with sliced ginger

Dinner
- Grass-fed or organic roast leg of lamb
- Steamed collards or kale topped with lemon and butter
- Wild rice
- Mixed fruit salad
- Glass tomato juice, salt and pepper

Day 11

Breakfast
- Oat bran cereal topped with Nutri-Sense; add cream or whole milk plus raw honey, nuts, and seeds.
- Organic turkey, chicken, or venison sausages (nitrate-free)
- Glass fresh-squeezed orange juice

Lunch
- Nut butter sandwich on coarse whole grain bread; spread on butter and honey, if desired
- Mixed greens salad topped with sliced turnips and radishes; drizzle with extra virgin olive oil and vinegar

Supper
- Grilled organic beefsteak, any type
- Grilled or raw onions
- Leftover wild rice
- Mixed vegetables, steamed
- Pomegranate Surprise

Day 12

Breakfast
- Nut butters (but not peanut) on cheese and vegetables
- 1/2 cantaloupe or honeydew melon
- Hot herbal tea with or without raw honey

Lunch
- Baked wild salmon or halibut (note: take a dropperful of the GreensFlush to detoxify the mercury)
- Steamed or boiled spinach
- Sliced papaya and kiwi
- Hot ginger tea

Supper

- Hamburger (organic/grass-fed source) and vegetable casserole; top with cheese, if desired
- Baked squash topped with nut butter or real butter; add cinnamon (squash is high in potassium and pro-vitamin A, that is beta carotene)

Day 13

Breakfast

- Nutri-Sense Super-Enriched Shake
  (mix 3 heaping tablespoons Nutri-Sense with whey protein shake and organic yogurt. Add a handful sunflower seeds or pine nuts. Add also raw honey and berries; blend, adding water to desired thickness)
- Ground buffalo or venison patty (sprinkle with OregaMax)
- Glass grapefruit juice or Pomegranate Surprise

Lunch

- Mixed green salad topped with salmon or sardines
- Oven-baked potatoes topped with parsley and spices
- Lemon or lime water

Supper

- Organic sirloin steak, medium or medium-rare
- Baked sweet potato topped with crude naturally pressed pumpkinseed oil (i.e. Pumpkinol) or nut butter
- Tossed salad with extra radishes and turnips (the latter provide selenium for immune protection plus antiseptic sulfur compounds); top with extra virgin olive oil and vinegar
- Herbal tea

Day 14

Breakfast

- 3 eggs over easy or poached
- Bowl oat bran cereal topped with Nutri-Sense, sliced almonds, and raw honey (i.e. wild oregano honey)
- Glass fresh-squeezed grapefruit juice

Lunch

- Salmon salad with diced vegetables, artichokes, cherry tomatoes, and olives (mix in crude pumpkinseed oil, i. e. Pumpkinol, and balsamic vinegar)
- Bowl Greek olives
- V-8 juice

Supper

- Lobster or crab legs (high in protein, fish oils, selenium, and zinc); drawn butter; lemon wedges
- Steamed mixed vegetables
- Tossed dark green salad with spicy greens like watercress, mustard greens, and arugula (top with extra virgin olive oil and lemon juice); add feta cheese, if desired
- Wedge melon or pineapple (note: the latter has antiseptic enzymes, but only when fresh)

Now you have it. These are special menus, which help the body kill germs. Plus, these foods strengthen cellular health, greatly increasing the resistance against disease. There is plenty of protein in these menus, which is needed for cellular strength and repair. The food is nutrient-dense, which greatly increases overall resistance. Regarding meat sources the selection of organic and grass-fed sources is crucial. For fish only the wild type must be eaten. By selecting healthy meats this will reduce the infection load placed upon the body. Regarding milk products and eggs it is crucial to consume only organic sources.

For an infection crisis or when a plague strikes, resistance is the difference between disease and health, in fact, life and death. The need for increased resistance is paramount. People are dying, and little is being done about it. Through the powers of nature and proper healthy diet innumerable lives could be saved. Peoples' health is being systematically degraded. Toxins of all sorts have overwhelmed the human body, greatly diminishing its powers. Today, people are suffering from a wide range of chronic diseases, largely due to weakened immunity. Yet, the health of the masses could be dramatically improved, strictly by making radical changes in the diet and by taking the appropriate nutritional supplements.

The power of pomegranate

The pomegranate is a special fruit with a history all its own. It is perhaps the most ancient citrus fruit, famous since the beginning of time for its health benefits. The Qur'an mentions it as a special fruit. Now it is known that of all fruit tested pomegranate scores the highest in antioxidant potential. It contains a greater amount of cell-protective antioxidants than any known fruit.

Pomegranate Syrup (North American Herb & Spice Co.) is a special kind of extract. It is made using the entire pomegranate by a unique process, which concentrates its potent flavonoids. The molasses is derived from a slow cooking process; a tablespoon of the syrup is equal to eating two or more of the fruit. What's more, the type of fruit is crucial. The syrup is derived from mountain-raised pomegranates, which largely grow wild. These pomegranates grow on mineral-rich rocky soil. Thus, these fruit, and, therefore, the syrup derived from them, are superior to the commercial type. This is the natural source of the pomegranate, which is why the Pomegranate Syrup has a unique sour taste, plus there is a flavonoid-rich residue, a thick natural 'mud' at the bottom of each bottle, which demonstrates its true nutrient density.

Use the Pomegranate Syrup on all meat dishes; it improves both flavor and digestion, plus it is protective. Add it to any citrus juice for a unique taste. Drizzle a small amount into organic yogurt or on cheese. For a dazzling taste add it to any stir-fry. It is an ideal marinade for fish of all types, especially salmon and char.

The flavonoids of pomegranate are mildly antiseptic. Plus, they protect the body from the noxious effects of heating, that is in relation to cooking meat. Use it liberally in any cooked dish. The molasses in particular helps prevent digestive distress, especially from heavy or meat dishes. A tablespoon or two in a glass of sparkling water makes the ideal after-dinner drink. As a result of consumption of this sumptuous food your health will significantly benefit. Pomegranate has a direct action for protecting the heart and arteries.

Chapter 7
Preventive Medicine

With dangerous germs preventing outbreaks is critical. Every means possible should be applied to avoid getting infections. The fact is improved hygienic habits play an enormous role in disease prevention. There are numerous procedures to follow in order to remain healthy. Thus, there is much that can be done to prevent the spread of disease.

Incredibly, the majority of diseases are preventable. It is far from inevitable to get sick. Measures can be taken, and sicknesses can be aborted. The key is to take action. A wait-and-see attitude is catastrophic and will result in the needless loss of life.

It is well known that disease is preventable. Hippocrates espoused this, as did the great 9th and 10th century Islamic masters, ar-Razi and Ibn Sina. The latter, along with Hippocrates, wrote extensively about the prevention of disease. R. L. Alsaker, writing in 1925, claimed that people truly "suffer needlessly and die prematurely" due to preventable infectious diseases. He claimed that in regard to respiratory afflictions in particular "it is easy to prevent or cure them."

In the early 20th century doctors had the ideal opportunity to study respiratory diseases: the flu pandemic. They saw untold millions of patients, taking histories, evaluating symptoms, examining tissues, and dispensing therapies. Many of these physicians determined that death from such infections was far from inevitable: it depended upon the resistance of the individual. If a person's tissues were already compromised, that is in the 1920s lingo, "if their blood and digestion were sick", they would succumb. If they had "healthy blood and digestion", they would survive. Using colds as an example Alsaker writes that the word itself is a misnomer. "Catching cold", he claims, is a misleading statement. While a cold is a type of inflammation of the respiratory tract these early doctors determined that the true origin of the sickness is within the tissues; the microbe itself cannot be blamed. Alsaker says further:

> "The cold manifests in the mucous membrane, but it is not a disease of the mucous membrane; the mucous membrane manifestations are only symptoms. A cold is a disease of the blood and digestive organs. To be more explicit, it is an indication that the digestion and the blood are deranged."

Alsaker then makes a dramatic claim:

> "Those who keep their digestive organs and their bloodstream in good condition never develop colds."

As has been demonstrated by doctors since ancient times becoming sick with common infections is far from inevitable. The majority of human afflictions are preventable. Good, solid hygienic and dietary habits prevent disease. People can take advantage of ancient and modern wisdom to stay healthy and even regain their health. Thus, it is possible to take advantage of the wisdom of the ancients combined with modern science to have a healthier, happier life. Let us learn how to take care of the self. This is the ideal "cure" for human ailments. Yet, always remember, "Good habits result in good health".

One way to keep the digestive tract in top condition is to take GreensFlush drops regularly. Simply take 10 to 20 drops twice daily to keep the gut, as well as bloodstream, in ideal condition. This nourishes, as well as cleanses, these tissues.

Dietary habits

What we eat and, in fact, fail to eat, has an enormous impact upon immunity. Poor dietary habits are perhaps the major cause of chronic disease. Thus, the diet has an enormous influence on the health of the blood, since this 'organ' consists largely of immune cells. What a person eats directly influences the health of the blood cells as well as the internal organs. This is what people fail to consider. The cells and organs of the body are directly influenced by the diet. They are made up of what a person eats. If the food is sick, that is toxic, so will be the blood cells and organs.

Food selections can predispose a person to serious or life-threatening infections. Heavily refined foods, such as pastries, doughnuts, pies, cakes, cupcakes, candy, white bread, white flour-based pastas, and soda pop, disrupt immunity. Certain of these foods, notably sugary sweets, high sugar pastries, cakes, pies, and/or soda pop, essentially stall immune activity, leaving the body wide open for infectious attacks. In Alsaker's terminology, as written in his book, *Curing Catarrh, Coughs, and Colds*, such foods disrupt the digestive system and pollute the blood. If the blood is polluted and the digestion disturbed, disease sets in. The fact is sugary sweets are so noxious that the consumption of such foods directly poisons the white blood cells, preventing them from performing their functions. In some instances such foods directly destroy the white cells, causing them to explode. Recent studies document how as little as a teaspoonful of sugar is enough to prevent white blood cells from performing their most critical function: phagocytosis, which means the destruction of germs. In other words, the sugar stalls white blood cell function, leaving the body vulnerable to germ attack.

Sugar is far from the only immune poison. Refined fats, nitrates and heated fats also damage it. The refined vegetable oils used in deep frying are particularly noxious. To quickly regain health avoid all deep fried foods or foods containing processed/refined vegetable oils. When such foods are eaten, the body absorbs the oils, incorporating them into the cells. Here, they poison the cells, leading to inflammation and suppressed immunity. Thus, the consequence of regularly eating heavily processed foods may be dire.

When the body is poisoned, it produces mucous, which breeds disease. Germs more readily gain a foothold. The individual develops a sort of mucousy disposition: the eyes water, the nose runs, the ears are plugged or drain, and the sinuses are stuffy or runny. The nose is runny and there are sneezing fits, hay fever and perhaps headache. All these symptoms may be produced by eating processed foods. The fact is these are the symptoms which occur typically in the fast food generation. Thus, these are signs of toxicity, not merely allergy. What's more, it demonstrates, as Alsaker says, that "sickness is a bad habit, not a necessity." Further, he notes that rather than purely external diseases it is the internal climate that accounts for the vulnerability to colds and flu. People who eat improperly are the primary victims. This is an incredible yet realistic statement. In other words, is it possible to essentially immunize the self against potentially fatal infections as well as bothersome cold/flu symptoms, just by eating right? In my experience this is largely the case, and this is precisely the approach described in Chapter 6.

Improper diet creates great toxicity within the system. The entire digestive system stalls, and toxins accumulate. These toxins cause the production of mucous, which further contaminates the system. The mucous builds up, weakening the system and making it vulnerable to germ attack. What's more, as a result of the accumulation of toxins the tissues become inflamed, which greatly weakens them. Such weakened tissue can be readily attacked by germs, especially the pandemic types. The inflammation, swelling, and toxicity, if unchecked, damage the tissues, causing cell death. This further weakens the organs and/or immune system, allowing germ invasion. Unless the excessive mucous and toxins are cleansed, the body will break down. The greater the amount of excess mucous in the body the more likely it is for germ attack. Mucous breeds germ growth, as it is the ideal medium, providing nourishment and a hiding place. As a result of the excess mucous chronic infections and even cancer become established. If the body is kept in balance by healthy eating practices and avoiding mucous-producing foods, there will be a high resistance against disease. A healthy, strong body, nourished by the proper toxin-free diet, will resist the most vile of infections, whereas the sickened body, overloaded with toxins and excessive mucous, will succumb.

The value of fasting

Numerous authors report that fasting strengthens immunity. Regular fasting reportedly increases lifespan. In fact, this makes sense. Occasional fasting allows the overworked systems to rest, especially the digestive organs. This digestive tract is constantly being stimulated, especially through the typical three-meal-a-day diet. Thus, through fasting the digestive tract, which is constantly bombarded with insults, is allowed to regenerate.

Digestion occupies a high percentage of the energy used by the body. Resting the digestive tract conserves body energy for more critical uses such as building the immune system, synthesis of critical compounds, and repair. The constant intake of food overwhelms the digestive system, leading to toxicity. Mucous accumulates, as does sludge, further weakening the system. People develop allergies, reactions, infections, and become overall weak. Their systems heal poorly and they are unable to easily recover. This clearly demonstrates the value of abstinence. Mere fasting from food, even without any other medicine, often revives health. It does so by allowing the body's own healing mechanisms to perform the cure. This is the immense benefit of fasting. The resting of the gut and the entire body is unmatched as a healing aid. Thus, fasting allows the body to cleanse itself. By continuously eating food the body has no opportunity to self cleanse. It becomes overloaded by the bulk of the food itself.

The original system for fasting was established by the Prophet Muhammad, about 620 A.D. Certainly, Christ preached fasting, performing it resolutely, as did Moses, Abraham, and numerous others. Yet, the deliberate system for fasting, which was later popularized by European physicians, owes its origin to Islam. Done properly this is a highly effective fast. It helps rest the gut allowing the body to heal itself. Yet, all the great men and women of earlier times, all spiritual sages, fasted. Many of them were reported to have lived a relatively long life, perhaps one hundred years or more. Certainly, fasting can largely be attributed for this incredible longevity. By resting the gut the human being will be healthier and will live longer. That is the prophetic guarantee.

The role of undernutrition

This is similar to fasting. Yet, it represents a more regular habit. It is the daily conscious effort to reduce calories. This is the most important tactic to decreasing disease, while increasing lifespan. What's more, as people age their caloric needs decline. It is simply not as crucial to eat huge amounts for the aging body. It was the Prophet Muhammad who said that the majority of diseases are due to the "stomach", that is to dietary indiscretions. Regarding the majority of these overeating takes precedence.

The stomach is a relatively small organ. It can readily be overwhelmed by excessive amounts of food. Eating smaller portions will result in health improvement, especially in the aged. At about 50 years of age the nutritional needs of the body decline significantly. Portions should be reduced. Food should be carefully and slowly chewed. Eating should never occur during excitement or for mere entertainment. For instance, eating while watching TV should be avoided.

Alsaker describes the dire results of overnutrition. The excessive food cannot be digested or processed. The food putrefies, creating toxicity. These poisons disrupt metabolism, leading to sickness. It is easy to avoid such internal poisoning: simply cut back on the total quantity of food. This will allow the digestive tract to deal with its burdens, giving it time to expel any toxins and residues. If the body is overloaded with additional food while it is toxic, then it is unable to process what it already contains. During any illness it is crucial to rest the gut. It must be allowed time to heal and cleanse. Undernutrition aids overall health as well as speeding recovery, that is from acute infections. This is accomplished by making a conscious effort to reduce the intake of solid foods. The body can more readily tolerate liquids such as juices and broths. It needs its energy to fight the infection. This is a simple formula for undernutrition.

The importance of blood-cleansing

Doctors of old stressed that if a person is sick, their blood is also sick. They realized that toxic blood weakened the constitution, making people vulnerable to the onset of disease. Thus, to be in optimal health the blood must be occasionally cleansed.

Natural medicines are potent blood cleansers. Drugs poison the blood. So do synthetic food additives. Toxic foods, such as processed meats, refined sugar, refined flour, and deep-fried foods, greatly upset blood chemistry.

The bloodstream, as well as, in fact, all the tissues, can be cleansed. One of the most potent remedies to do so is the wild greens extract known as GreensFlush. This is a wild raw greens concentrate, which is unlike any other. It is wild bush greens with potent cleansing properties, including wild dandelion and burdock. A potent tissue, liver, and blood cleanser this is the ideal tonic for detoxification. People who take it gain significant health benefits. These benefits include greater vigor, more strength, improved digestion, a healthier immune system, and improved appearance. This is because GreensFlush helps purge noxious poisons from the organs and blood. It is because of this mechanism that it improves overall health. The GreensFlush can only be ordered by mail: 1-800-243-5242.

The cells of the body readily become toxic. They do so just from normal aging. To halt this process the cells and organs must be constantly purged. What's more, if the blood is toxic, so will be the cells and organs. The wild greens is the ideal means to purge. It purges the toxins directly from the liver and the gut. Regular greens, that is wheat grass, barley grass, and other "farmed" products, fail to create such a power. While they do contain a degree of cleansing power, they lack the tremendous potency of wild-growing greens, which are far more aggressive in their ability to purge poisons.

Certain spice extracts are blood-cleansing. They exert this action by purging the liver of toxins. Enzyme synthesis within the liver is also bolstered. LivaClenz formula is an ideal addition to any blood-cleansing plan. It dramatically improves liver function, aiding in the removal of toxins. This results in improved appearance, stronger immunity, and improved digestion. The fact is through the regular intake of this supplement there is a pleasant side effect: naturally improved or normalized bowel function.

Cigarette smoking and alcohol

There is no question that smokers and drinkers are at a heightened risk for a variety of diseases. Both alcohol and tobacco depress the immune system, increasing the vulnerability to serious conditions. Tobacco smokers are at a high risk for communicable respiratory infections. Tobacco smoke greatly depresses the immune system of the lungs, especially the cilia. The latter are the lungs' cleansing apparatus, sort of their street cleaner. Cigarette smoke paralyzes the cilia, allowing germs to easily infect the lungs. This is a diabolical habit. It damages not only the smoker but also all who are nearby. Even from a distance it creates toxicity: a smoker who is in a car can cause toxicity to others just through the tobacco residues on his or her clothes. Smoking kills not only the smokers but also innocent bystanders, including close relatives and even children. The fact is thousands of individuals die every year as a consequence of secondhand smoke.

Residues from cigarettes can be purged. This may be achieved through a combination approach of the potent spice extracts plus the GreensFlush. Take the Oregacyn, two capsules twice daily, along with the oil of oregano, five to ten drops under the tongue several times daily. Also, take the GreensFlush, 40 drops under the tongue twice daily.

Coffee, hot tea, and iced tea

These beverages are superior to the 'synthetic' drinks such as soda pop and artificially colored fruit drinks. Yet, if they are consumed to an excess, they can aggravate or even cause illness.

American physicians practicing in the early 20th century found that the excessive intake of coffee and tea, especially if taken with sugar, lowered overall resistance. Tea itself possesses immune-benefitting properties. However, it is a strong diuretic and, therefore, may cause the depletion of certain nutrients, including rather critical ones such as vitamin C, magnesium, potassium, and folic acid. Black tea leaves also destroy thiamine, and the regular intake of this beverage can induce this deficiency. Symptoms of thiamine deficiency are numerous and include premature graying of the hair, muscle weakness, fatigue, rapid heart rate, numbness and tingling, nerve pain, nervousness, mood swings, depression, anxiety, fears, paranoia, personality changes, insomnia, nightmares, and anger.

It is easy to understand from this list of symptoms why thiamine is known as the "morale vitamin". Thus, Dr. Alsaker correctly observed that anything consumed in excess, even natural black tea, can disrupt body chemistry, leaving the individual vulnerable to disease. For those who drink black tea it should be limited to a cup or two per day. Drink it with real whole milk and raw honey instead of sugar. Iced tea is even more aggressive in depleting key nutrients. If sweetened with aspartame it becomes a bona fide toxin, disrupting the chemistry of all cells. Aspartame itself destroys nutrients, notably thiamine, folic acid, and vitamin C. Thus, iced tea, sweetened artificially, greatly depletes key nutrients, particularly vitamin C, folic acid, and thiamine. No wonder that deafness and neurological disorders, which are symptoms of extreme thiamine deficiency, are so common in aspartame users.

Chocolate, cocoa, and hot chocolate

Chocolate suppresses the immune system, especially if it is laced with sugar. People become readily addicted to chocolate, eating vast quantities. They may even develop an allergy to it.

Allergic intolerance greatly depresses the immune system. This may result in depressed white blood cell activity, which sets the stage for infection. During epidemic times a person needs as much immune reserve as possible. Thus, it is important to avoid any potentially allergenic foods. Allergy to chocolate may result in a wide range of symptoms, including headache, stuffy sinuses, bronchial congestion, sinus pressure, migraines, depression, mood swings, cold sore outbreaks, digestive disturbances, back pain, and nervousness.

Cocoa and chocolate are stimulants. Such stimulants deplete nutrients from the body. Plus, by agitating the nervous system, as well as the adrenal glands, they weaken the body. This is how they increase the vulnerability to infection. For a more powerful immune system avoid the excessive consumption of cocoa or chocolate. A light dusting of cocoa powder over warm milk or fruit is harmless. However, the addictive consumption of it in large quantities greatly suppresses immune function. What's more, if a person is allergic to it, which may be manifested by sinus problems, headaches, agitation, depression, anxiety, and digestive disorders, it must be strictly avoided.

Carnivorous animals: death in waiting

Carnivorous animals breed disease. They eat diseased animals, such as rats and mice, as well as sick or weakened prey, and are contaminated with disease-breeding germs within their tissues. Thus, anyone who eats such animals will acquire their diseases.

Such animals may be involved in the SARS outbreak. Evidence indicates that certain viruses, known as coronaviruses, found in animals of the rodent family, such as the civet cat and raccoon, may cause this disease. The Chinese eat such animals, contracting the infection from the animal meat. The germs breed within the Chinese, developing the ability to infect them. Thus, the Chinese, who eat dangerous meats, act as a genetic brewery, allowing the jumping of species. The current SARS pandemic is thought to be due to the dire Asian habit of eating civet cats, an animal related to rodents. Such "cats" are held in pens in Chinese restaurants, cooked to order for unsuspecting patrons. Civet cats, a name which is a misnomer, since this animal is a type of mongoose—a type of rodent—harbor a wide range of aggressive viruses, including the coronavirus implicated in SARS. These viruses cause highly destructive diseases, including hemorrhagic fevers. The fact is virtually the exact coronavirus implicated as a cause of SARS has been found in such cats. It would be no surprise if such a virus was originally rodent in origin, since mice are a major part of the civet cat's, or, rather, rodent's, diet.

Civet cats are inedible. Eating them will lead to a variety of diseases. Efforts should be made to halt such practices. Tame or caged civet cats must be destroyed and their consumption prohibited. The Asian habit of eating animals from the rodent family, such as civet cats and other mongoose-like creatures, will result in incredible rates of disease. Plus, this will cause the dissemination of worldwide plagues, which will sicken and kill untold millions of people. SARS itself is a rodent-like plague, that is the germ is certainly rodent in origin. Rodent genes have been found in the viral sequence of the SARS virus. It behaves like a plague, that is it is highly contagious. Like the plague it sickens people quickly, killing a high percentage.

In my earlier book, *The Respiratory Solution* (Revised Edition), I predicted that regarding the SARS epidemic the consumption of rodents was largely the cause. This was recently confirmed by the WHO (January 2004), when they claimed that, in fact, the virus infecting humans is the same as the one found in rodents. The fact is people who sold, that is handled, these rodents were among the disease's first victims, which I also predicted. Thus, *The Respiratory Solution* preempts the WHO.

Certainly, it is highly unhealthy to eat rats or any other animal from the rodent family. By eating rodents the stage is set for the development of international plagues. This is because regardless of cooking a number of rodent-source germs will survive, multiplying within the body. Such germs may develop the critical "species jump", and, thus, develop into a full-fledged human germ. Yet, incredibly, despite the seemingly obvious dangers certain Asians, in fact, hunt rats, eating them as a prize. Animals in this family include squirrels, rats, mice, mongoose, opossums, civet cats, and raccoons. These animals breed a vast number of diseases. They are scavengers, and they eat carrion. Common sense would indicate that they are inedible.

Many Americans are unaware of the dangers of eating such animals. Consider squirrel hunters. They eat this meat, which tastes somewhat like chicken, thinking they are eating relatively safe food. Yet, they fail to realize that squirrels are rodents and, therefore, they transmit rodent-like diseases.

The flesh from such animals is ridden with disease-causing parasites, many of which resist death from normal cooking temperatures. A number of these parasites are encysted, meaning they survive heat. After consumption of the meat, the cysts are broken down by stomach acid, ultimately releasing the parasite. If this parasite survives the digestive process, it multiplies, infecting the intestines. From here it may invade through the intestinal wall into the bloodstream to infect blood cells or internal organs. No organ is immune, but most parasites prefer the intestines, lungs, and/or liver as the primary sites for infection. The fact is in people with chronic brain diseases, including CJD, germs derived from rodents have been found, including the rodent-source spirochetes.

Pork: a major cause of disease

All holy books prohibit the consumption of pork flesh. Christ prohibited it, as did Moses. Originally, the Bible prohibited it, although, today, this prohibition is largely forgotten. A more recent holy book, that is the Qur'an, also prohibits its consumption. There must be a reason for this.

Why would the great prophets emphasize its prohibition? Why would the holy books condemn it? Certainly, a single mere parasitic illness, trichinosis, would fail to fully explain it. There must be other factors.

The reasoning is rather simple. Pigs are omnivores, that is they eat a varied diet. This diet includes animal foods, including carrion. Pigs eat all varieties of wastes, including the feces of other animals. Like other flesh eaters, they breed a wide range of diseases. Pigs are the host of hundreds of parasitic infections. They also are infected with unique types of encysted bacteria and parasites. The cysts of these germs are impossible to destroy at normal cooking temperatures. Thus, pork flesh is unfit for human consumption. It is a contaminated flesh, which is impossible to render safe. I recall the time that a fellow medical school student dined at a picnic, which featured grilled bratwurst. Within 24 hours he became violently ill, suffering from severe intestinal cramps, diarrhea, chest pain, and back pain. Certainly, he contracted a porcine parasite, possibly trichinosis. As a result, his health was never the same.

The pork producers will be hostile at these words. Yet, this is irrefutable. The fact is the regular consumption of pork causes a wide range of symptoms and diseases, including arthritis, rheumatoid arthritis, esophageal swelling, chronic upper back pain, gallbladder spasms, gallstones, lupus, and pancreatitis. A variety of cancers are related to pork consumption, particularly stomach, esophageal, colon, and breast cancers. What's more, a recent report demonstrates an ominous finding: people who regularly eat ham have an increased risk for neurological diseases: in other words, mad cow-like syndromes. The fact is for regular or heavy ham eaters as described in the *Journal of Epidemiology* the risks for mad cow-like syndromes rises some 1000%.

Certainly, this is far from condemning the animal itself. It is merely the fact that the meat of this animal is unhealthy, regardless of how it is raised. This is because like all other meat-eating animals the flesh of pork is disease-spreading. Pigs harbor highly aggressive parasites, many of which are encysted. Cooking fails to destroy the cysts. When the meat is eaten, the cysts are weakened by stomach acid. Ultimately, they open, releasing the parasitic larvae or bacteria. These revived germs multiply, causing localized or systemic infection. Many of these parasites cause deep infection, leading to inflammation. Over time this aggression can induce cancer.

There is another reason pigs are dangerous: global pandemics. The majority of the worldwide flu infections, which killed millions of people, originated in them. In other words, swine were the original breweries. The viruses multiplied by the trillions in swine.

Through coughing and sneezing these animals disseminated these germs, which then infected farmers and others nearby. Infected humans act as super-infectors, spreading the disease throughout the rest of the population. Thus, megafarming of pigs is far from a mere "economic right": it is a highly deadly practice, which places the entire human race at risk. The Malaysian experience fully demonstrated this. Here, the potential risks of intensive pig farming were proven firsthand. A devastating influenza virus struck, destroying peoples' nervous systems. A third of those infected died, the primary victims being pig farmers. It was directly traced to sick pigs in huge pig cities. Tens of thousands of pigs were slaughtered, and, thus, the spread of this disease was halted.

When pigs are infected with aggressive flu viruses, it is no pleasant scene. They develop a phenomenally powerful cough and/or sneeze, which is explosive. Thus, like a biological cannon they can spew germs far into the air, spreading them hundreds of feet away. The farmers become infected, as do passersby. These people become the progenitors of potentially deadly infections, feeding the germs into the rest of the population. Thus, it may be expected that any state harboring intensive pig farms will suffer severely in the coming flu pandemic. The fact is mass death can have its origin in a single pig farm. No wonder pork consumption is divinely prohibited. The fact is even the flesh is dangerous to consume, particularly in the midst of a flu pandemic.

Recently, in Ohio another swine-related disease has captured headlines. It is a vague condition afflicting people who live down-wind of intensive pig farms. The victims suffer from debilitating pain, arthritis, exhaustion, and unexplainable lung/bronchial symptoms. Their symptoms worsen whenever the wind is right, that is when it delivers the reeking stench. Doctors do not dispute that the people are sick. However, they are at a loss to explain the cause. The people are certain of it: it is the sickening air, which arises from the intensive pig farming. This pork farm air, teeming with microbes, is

inhaled. The smell alone sickens the individual. While humans abho
it, they usually fail to realize that the air may also be infective. Th
gases which are liberated from swine feces are also toxic, in fact
they suppress the immune system. Such gases, including methan
and sulfur dioxide, are among the most toxic known to humankind

Proper hand-washing

This is the most essential of all hygienic procedures. Proper hand
washing technique preserves health and saves lives. The fact is b
strictly adhering to such techniques potentially millions of live
could be saved every year.

Pump soaps are ideal for hand-washing. Bar soaps often bree
germs. This is because certain germs, in fact, thrive by eatin
soap residues, which are rich in organic material. If using ba
soaps, spray occasionally with Germ-a-Clenz. Add either oil o
wild oregano or Oregacyn Oil to pump soaps, about 3 droppersfu
per container. This will prevent the transmission of germs. Thi
"home chemistry" approach is far superior to relying upo
commercial antiseptic pump soaps, laced with syntheti
chemicals, fragrances, and dyes. In contrast to these commercia
types oil of oregano-fortified pump soaps fail to promot
dangerous microbial resistance. So, buy the healthiest pump soa
available and make your own antiseptic solution. This is far mor
hygienic than using chemical-based soaps or bar soaps. Use onl
edible oil of wild oregano (i.e. Oreganol): avoid the cheape
Thymus capitus and/or Origanum vulgare. The latter have neve
been proven safe. In contrast, oregano oil from the wild-growin
spice is fully safe, even in large amounts.

Here is the ideal hand-washing technique. Turn on the fauce
Pump one or two squirts of oregano-fortified pump soap. Using
small amount of water rub vigorously over the hands. Then, rins
thoroughly, leaving no residues of soap or suds. Dry the hand
thoroughly on a fresh towel.

Hand-washing reduces the incidence of disease astronomically. f a person is persistent in proper hand-washing hygiene, there is a significant reduction in infectious disease.

Showering

When showering, certain procedures may be followed, which will help improve overall health. First, wash the mouth and face, then the hair. Then, wash the rest of the body. Wash the privates last, i.e. after washing the head, hair, mouth, etc. Spread the buttocks and allow the water to cleanse the anus. For women always wash the anus from front to back. Dry the feet carefully after showering and also between the toes to prevent fungal growth. Spray feet before placing socks with Germ-a-Clenz or rub with oil of wild oregano.

Recently, certain dangers of showering have been noted. The hot steam causes germs to become volatilized, and, thus, they can be inhaled. This can be neutralized by spraying the Germ-a-Clenz about the shower before showering. There is another useful technique: simply squirt the Oreganol on the shower floor, and let it become volatilized by the hot steam. This will protect the lungs from the noxious effects of airborne germs and mold.

Toilet hygiene

Few people realize that there is an entire etiquette to proper toilet hygiene. In Japan a special effort is made for this procedure. In countries of high Muslim populations a special technique is followed, which is taught from childhood. Such procedures and techniques are worth investigating, that is for their disease-prevention benefits.

The Japanese have created elaborate toilets, which dispense a metered dose of water, often fortified with antiseptics or perfumes. Adopting the procedure from the Prophet Muhammad, people of the Islamic faith follow a specific method. This is in part to properly prepare the body for ritual worship. After all dribbling is exhausted, that is that no urine remains in the urethra, the genitals are rinsed to cleanse any residues. This reduces the transmission of infectiou diseases, plus it eliminates any odor. Through such a rinsing technique by men the fact is women are protected. This is because urine is an ideal medium for germ growth and if it is cleansed from the body, germ growth is reduced. What's more, Muslims, as well as Jews, retain the circumcision ritual. While controversy has been raised regarding it, from a disease-prevention point of view it is essential. Plus, there is good research which documents how failure to circumsize perpetuates disease, both in the male and in any sexual contacts. The prepuce breeds disease-causing germs, because it traps urine against the penile head. Urine is an ideal medium for growth. It is exceptionally difficult to adhere to proper hygiene with a foreskin. Invariably, germs hide on the surface between the skin and the penile head. In that dark environment they grow readily. These germs may migrate backwards, up into the urethra, prostate, bladder, and even into kidneys. This may explain the heightened incidence of prostate and kidney infections in uncircumcised men. Jesus was adamant about the need for circumcision. So was the prophet Muhammad. In the supposedly last gospel of Jesus, the so called Gospel of Barnabas, Jesus is quoted as saying that it is an act of Satan to remain uncircumcised. In other words, remaining uncircumcised leads to damaging consequences.

The public toilet requires special consideration. It is voluminously contaminated with germs. The seats contain potentially billions of organisms. Sitting directly on the seat may cause infection. The buttocks may readily become infected, but so can the genitals. However, it is rare to contract venereal disease from the seats, but it is far from impossible. Usually, the infections are more of an annoying nature, like boils and irritations. Even so, direct exposure to another person's germs is eviling. Would anyone in their right mind be intimate with what s essentially dozens of other peoples' wastes? This is done unthinkingly by millions of Americans every day. One obvious method of prevention is to line the toilet seat with tissue paper. This is a cumbersome technique, however, it is effective. Another method is to use an antiseptic spray such as Germ-a-Clenz. Simply spray the seat with the Germ-a-Clenz. Wipe dry with tissue, being careful not to touch the seat with bare hands. Then, the seat is safer to sit on. Another dilemma is splash. This occurs when hard stool hits the toilet water. The contaminated water splashes against the buttocks and genitals, potentially inoculating them with disease-causing germs. One way to minimize this is to do what may be discussed as an "anti-splash" technique. Simply add toilet paper to the center of the stool water before using it. Do not use Kleenex or paper towels, as this will plug the toilet. This technique will minimize splash. If splash does occur, there is a simple solution: spray the area with Germ-a-Clenz. Since no direct contact is necessary this is highly hygienic. This helps neutralize any contaminate, but it does burn mildly temporarily. Avoid spraying directly on the genitals. If this must be done, be aware of a temporary but harmless burning sensation.

The air in public restrooms is foul. This can be resolved with the Germ-a-Clenz. Upon entering the restroom pump a few sprays high into the air. After entering the stall spray above and let drift down. This may also be done regularly in home restrooms to both eliminate odors and decontaminate germs. Every time a toilet is flushed millions of germs are disseminated into the air. After flushing mist with Germ-a-Clenz; this will help prevent the inhalation of noxious germs.

Household pets

This is a delicate subject for many people. Pets provide a great deal of love. In many respects they provide pleasure greater than many humans. Yet, the fact is household pets can transmit a wide range of diseases. Certain types of pets represent a greater risk than others, for instance, dogs. This is no condemnation of such animals. It is strictly a biological fact. Dogs carry highly virulent viruses, as well as parasites, which may readily infect humans. The viruses found in dog saliva have been directly linked to a number of illnesses, including lupus, rheumatoid arthritis, scleroderma, fibromyalgia, and cancer. Cats are considerably safer, largely because they keep a relative distance from humans. Plus, cats are fastidious about hygiene. However, they too may transmit various germs. Yet, other than cat scratch fever no major human disease has been associated with domestic cats.

It is the saliva of dogs which is exceptionally dangerous. This is because this saliva contains a wide variety of viruses, capable of causing human diseases. Canine salivary viruses are highly aggressive, and can attack and infest any internal organ. In this respect they are readily able to cause cell death. The fact is they are stealth viruses and thus, readily evade the immune system. The majority of such diseases are chronic. Usually, other than perhaps a sore throat or flu-like illness no acute symptoms are noticed. Dog saliva and, particularly, feces, may also contain the cysts of worms such as the canine heartworm. Incredibly, there are thousands of cases of Americans who are infected with canine heartworm.

Many of the diseases contracted from dogs are wasting diseases, the result of the gradual decay of human cells from the aggressive invasion of canine stealth viruses. Many of these viruses have a predilection for the nervous system, that is the brain and spinal cord. The neurological diseases which may be caused by canine stealth viruses include multiple sclerosis, ALS (Lou Gehrig's disease), Parkinson's disease, various types of dementia, and Alzheimer's disease.

One way to minimize the virulence of canine salivary viruses is to attempt to reduce the levels of these viruses within the tissues

his may be done both in an infected human and the host. While it
may not be possible to completely destroy them, certainly, their
evels can be reduced. The fact is such viruses may serve a type of
ymbiotic function within the animal. Therefore, an attempt to
sterilize" them may be inappropriate. However, by keeping their
evels down, certainly, the health of the animal will improve. This
may be achieved through the intake of antiseptic spice oils. Among
hese the Oregacyn multiple oil complex is ideal. This formula
ontains several antiviral spice oils, plus it contains oil of wild
umin, a highly aggressive antiparasitic agent. Dogs carry a wide
ange of parasites, which may also infect humans. As an antiviral
nd antiparasitic purge give the dog oil of Oregacyn, 2 to 5 or
nore drops twice daily. Higher doses are acceptable for large
ogs, for instance, 5 to 10 drops twice daily.

Reptiles are yet another source of invasive microbes. They
ransmit both parasites and bacteria. Reptiles transmit a novel
ype of salmonella, which can infect humans, causing diarrhea
nd abdominal distress. Such pets must be handled with caution
nd any handling necessitates vigorous hygiene, that is careful
ashing. Unless hands are washed after handling reptiles human
nfection is inevitable. To reduce the transmission of reptilian
iseases spray the air about the cage with Germ-a-Clenz. Add a
rop of oil of Oregacyn to the drinking water. Note: the oil of
Oregacyn may be added to the water of any pet to keep bacteria,
iral, and parasitic counts down, both in the water and animal.

Birds may transmit certain bacteria and fungi. Commonly,
ird droppings are contaminated with germs, which, if becoming
irborne, can infect humans. There is a simple solution: oil of
ild oregano and Germ-a-Clenz. Simply spray the latter about
he cage; let mist drift downward. Add a drop of oil of oregano
o drinking water. Birds take this well. The oil helps prevent
arious avian flu infections as well as avian pneumonia. Pet
hops are currently using the oil successfully to prevent lung

infections in commercial birds. For pet shop owners the Germ-a Clenz, when sprayed in the shop, eliminates odors and destroy potentially dangerous germs. Because of the dust, fec contaminants, organic matter, and dander, the air in pet shops potentially poisonous. The plethora of organic matter breed germs. This can be safely neutralized through the misting spic oils. Misting the Germ-a-Clenz should be a daily routine in p shops or in homes housing large amounts of pets.

Proper exercise

Regular exercise is crucial for optimal health to achieve this. It unnecessary to do combative sports or aggressive weight liftin, Rather, simple, non-aggressive exercises will suffice. The ide exercise is brisk walking. Incredibly, brisk walking burns mo energy than jogging. Swimming and bicycling are also excelle exercises. These are the best choices for the average individual

There is another benefit of exercise. It forces the person breathe, since the body demands oxygen for metabolism. Thu during exercise there is a need for deep or clear breathing, whic helps not only deliver more oxygen to the body but also helps th body expel waste gases trapped deep within the lungs.

Deep breathing

There is an art to proper breathing. Incredibly, today people mu make a conscious effort to breathe properly. This is becau: people are enduring such excessive stress that this affects the breathing. Plus, the air is foul. What's more, people spend mo of their time indoors, and fresh air is a rare commodity.

Impure air is a significant cause of disease. The air in majc cities is dangerous, especially near major highways and airport Especially in the winter or late fall the constant intake of impui indoor air can, in fact, cause or certainly aggravate colds or flu.

Make a concerted effort to breathe deeply. Feel the chest expand. Ideally, breathe from the lower part of the abdomen, even pelvis, not from the chest. Attempt to determine which emotions are restricting your breathing. Anger, apathy, and frustration restrict breathing. Eliminate such emotions.

Sunlight

Adequate sunlight is crucial for overall health. Yet, there is a balance in this. Excessive sunlight or sudden exposure to the hot sun can depress immunity. Thus, there is a balance in everything. To benefit from the sun the exposure must be regular and gradual. Avoid the noon sun. The ideal time for exposure is from mid-morning to about 11:00 a.m. and from about 3:00 p.m. until just before sunset. A half hour or hour twice daily is sufficient exposure. Sunbathing is not advised, that is unless it is done in short bursts of one half hour to one hour maximum.

Water

The body is mostly water. If the water in the body is impure, all organs will suffer. Thus, if the water that is consumed is contaminated, the body will become contaminated.

Globally, water-borne illnesses are the primary cause of death and disability. In the Third World it is these illnesses which account for the extensive occurrence of disability, devastation, and death. The fact is tens of millions of people die every year as a consequence of the consumption of contaminated water.

To remain in optimal health the individual must be vigilant about drinking water. A person can be readily poisoned by water, even if it appears crystal clear. Thus, in order to maintain excellent health the issue of the quality of the water must be resolved. Water can poison in many ways. This is because water is a solvent; it can actually transport poisons into the body. It can

do so both through ingestion as well as topically. Studies prov
that merely washing, bathing, or showering in toxic water leads 1
the absorption of impurities: directly through the skin. What
more, while tap water might appear to be relatively sterile, it is f₂
from safe. The fact is due to its high chlorine content it suppresse
the immune system. Incredibly, tap water contains a wide range c
highly poisonous compounds: known carcinogens. Plu
increasingly, it contains high levels of drugs, residues from huma
and animal intake. The drugs may remain active in water for yea
and, thus, are constantly recycled in the water table. Toxic levels c
drugs are thought responsible for the high rate of cancer in peop
who drink tap water. Certain of such drugs, notably estrogens ar
other hormones, are directly correlated with a bizarre conditio
premature development in children. The fact is there is a virtu
epidemic of premature sexual development, as well as childhoc
obesity, which is directly tied to estrogenic drugs. The drugs appe₂
in the waterways through the urine and feces of humans as well ₂
animals. Such drugs are invisible poisons. Every effort should t
made to remove them from drinkable water.

Only pure water, free of chemicals, as well as germs, can kee
the immune system in ideal condition. Water can be purifie
through machines or other devices. Also, high quality bottle
waters can be procured. Distillation may remove the majority c
toxins, but it also removes invaluable minerals. Plus, distille
water is a solvent, that is it depletes minerals from the bod
Reverse osmosis is another commonly used method. Howeve
this method also causes vast mineral losses. Research h₂
documented how soft water is associated with an increased ris
for stroke as well as heart attacks. The consumption of suc
water also increases the risks for cancer. Thus, the use c
distilled or reverse osmosis water is inadvisable.

A high quality tap water purification system is available. Know
as Lifesource Water Purification Systems this is an activated carbc

method of the highest quality. Using a state-of-the-art technology his company specializes in whole house units, although smaller apartment-sized systems are available. The units are tested and certified by NSF, making the Lifesource unit the only such system available. Lifesource specializes only in home and apartment water treatment units, offering award winning technology. This is the type of unit I have in my home. In fact, I can safely use the water in my home for bathing, cooking, and drinking. The Lifesource unit is truly a high grade system, which is guaranteed. It removes the vast majority of contaminants, while converting the water to a pleasant tasting and nourishing form. Protect your family from the ominous danger of invisible contaminants, which can cause outright diseases: cancer, heart disease, high blood pressure, premature sexuality, infertility, thyroid disorders, senility disorders, and untold other sicknesses.

This system is ideal for people who own their houses. It will safely and efficiently remove the contaminants that place a person's life at risk. The contaminants in water are fulminant carcinogens, which are readily absorbed through the skin. What's more, their harsh actions can initiate internal cancers, especially colon and rectal cancers. All this can be prevented by proper in-home water treatment, which the Lifesource unit readily achieves. By installing this system within the home the health of the entire family will benefit. Plus, the risks for degenerative disease, particularly cancer, arthritis, and heart disease, will significantly decline. For more information contact a sales rep at:

Lifesource Water Purification Systems
123 S. Fair Oaks Ave
Pasadena, California
1-800-992-3997
Web Site: www.lifesourcewater.com

Chapter 8
Saving Lives

ll other books about pandemics and/or epidemics expose the
oblem. In other words, they all warn of impending doom. Only
is book explains what action to take. Only this book provides
e cures. It is possible to avoid the horrors of killer infections.
his can be achieved by regularly making use of natural cures
us boosting the immune system.

There are a wide range of killer pandemics, which are killing
ndreds of thousands of Americans yearly. Webster's defines a
ndemic as a disease occurring over a large region. This fully
plains the diseases of today: AIDS, SARS, hepatitis, bizarre flu
ndromes, chronic fatigue syndrome, Helicobacter pylori, Lyme,
d tuberculosis. Such diseases kill tens of millions globally every
ar and disable uncountable others. Yet, how many additional
ndemics can humanity withstand before it is crushed? Sickness
ay well ruin this race before any predicted divine intervention.
hese are sicknesses which humanity has itself caused. What's
ore, they are sicknesses which in many respects can be
versed, that is if we turn to nature.

There are no synthetic drugs for pandemics, nor can any drug
r surgery cure. Thus, to combat epidemics the only option is the

natural medicine chest. Here, there are hundreds of cures. Th
book merely describes the most readily available, as well as pote
of all cures. Plus, the cures described herein are utterly safe: the
is no possibility of serious side effects. Thus, these cures are id
for use in the event of widespread diseases, where the medi
system is overwhelmed and where people are largely left to th
own devices. In other words, if an individual is cut off fro
medical care these cures will prove invaluable. Yet, where does
person turn? The individual is seemingly overcome by potential
deadly germs. The body is readily infected by such germs, whi
cause slow, writhing infections. SARS, AIDS, West Nile, stap
strep, Norwalk, SV40, chlamydia, herpes, and drug-resista
germs, all are infecting the population. Americans are in a di
state. People are getting sick constantly, and they are unable
become cured. What's more, often, they lack the money to buy t
medicines they need. This is why home cures are so invaluable. F
a few cents per day an individual can stay well, or, in the event
illness, get well.

Hospitals are dangerous places. This is another reason wl
home cures are invaluable. In hospitals the air is foul and tl
surfaces contaminated. Each year new diseases emerge fro
them, largely a consequence of the overuse of potent medicine
in particular, antibiotics. Such medicines create mutated germ
freaks of nature, which readily infect humans. In other word
the overuse of these medicines leads to unique diseases nev
before known to humankind. These mutants cause uncountab
agony, pain, and misery as well as death. Such infections a
examples of human meddling; the excessive use of pote
antibiotics, which have caused this pandemic. The fact is son
250,000 people die in hospitals alone in the United States ea
year from such bizarre germs. This is the minimum number
deaths from drug-induced mutants. The number who die outsi
of hospitals is unknown but it must number in the tens

ousands. Globally, on a yearly basis millions of people die as result of antibiotic resistance. From a medical point of view the utations are incurable. Drugs only further aggravate the lemma. Only natural medicines offer hope for a cure. The fact recent data proves them curative. A study published by eorgetown University has shown that spice extracts, that is the reganol P73, destroy drug-resistant germs. Even penicillin-sistant staph succumbed. The Oreganol was nearly equal to a otent antibiotic, Vancomycin, in its ability to destroy drug-sistant germs, a stupendous result for a natural food.

The risk for such infections is dramatically rising. Many of these fections seem unstoppable. Modern medicine is impotent in ocking or even delaying their advance. Help must arise from other uarters. This is in the form of natural cures. The fact is natural cures verse disease, without serious side effects. In contrast, drugs are ajor killers, accounting for tens of thousands of deaths yearly. us, they cause extensive tissue and organ damage. This is the fference between truly natural cures and the synthetics.

The Being who created this universe is capable of doing ything, including providing potent cures which can reverse man diseases. Interestingly, it was the Prophet Muhammad who st said, "For every disease God has created its cure." What's ore, he added, if it is unknown, it is just that humanity has yet to discovered. Thus, on this planet there exists a cure for virtually ery disease. That demonstrates the tremendous consideration, as ell as love, of the divine being, that is for His creation.

Some people fail to believe in such a concept. Yet, careful nsideration of the issues will demonstrate its validity. The nthetic, that is man-made, chemicals have utterly failed to stem e tide of infectious diseases. What's more, such substances, in fact, ve caused a number of epidemics. Furthermore, the synthetics ve caused premature deaths. In contrast, natural compounds, that safe, edible substances, used in the treatment of disease have

never created epidemics. Nor have they caused significant pai
agony, and death. Rather, such substances save lives.

Natural remedies are highly complicated, and their chemic
structure cannot be totally discovered. Who made su
compounds? Why do they work within the human body witho
causing disease or death? Why do synthetic drugs cause hundre
of thousands of deaths every year, while natural herbs or toni
fail to cause them? Can anyone name even a single death from
pure or unprocessed herb or food extract? In a year or even ov
five or ten years is even a single such case recorded? This whi
according to the *JAMA* some 115,000 people die from the intal
of synthetic drugs, which are properly prescribed. This fails
include the deaths from drugs prescribed in error or those caus
by antibiotics, which are responsible for drug-resistant bacteri
and fungal infections. If all these are calculated, the total year
deaths reaches nearly 500,000, making it the second or thi
leading cause of death. How are such souls replaced? Is tl
anything but utter tyranny?

True, people can die from certain natural substances. Tho
who are allergic to certain foods, such as peanuts, can die fro
shock. Yet, the fact is it is virtually unheard of for a natural her
such as garlic, onion, oregano, echinacea, etc., to cause ev
minor harm, let alone death. What's more, certainly, the numb
of cases of organ damage caused by such substances is nil if n
nonexistent. Truly, natural foods are the most harmless of a
substances. Medicines which are made from them should be t
first line of therapy.

Yet, something must be done. There is only apathy regardi
such diseases. Years after the outbreak no cures are found. Al
is decades old. There is no medical cure. Hepatitis C is regard
as incurable. No cures are available even for the common cold
flu. In the pharmaceutical world there is nothing to halt t
onslaught of drug-resistant germs. The fact is drugs created t

idemic. Thus, while medicines are causing diseases it is the natural medicines, the very medicines created by almighty God, which reverse them. Millions of Americans, who have been sickened by pharmaceutical agents, as well as vaccines, have benefitted from natural medicines. Plus, many such medicines have behind them a greater degree of research than many pharmaceuticals. A recent study at Georgetown University proves that, for instance, a special blend of wild oregano oils, known as Oreganol P73, destroyed drug-resistant germs. The point is there is no need to lose hope. Even though humankind, in its greed and lust for money and power, has caused vast debacles, the natural substances can save the day. In other words, by turning to natural medicines, that is the medicines which were created for human benefit: this is the best chance for survival.

The human medicines offer not even a single cure, not even hope. However, there are thousands of cures available in the natural pharmacy offering hope and ease for virtually every known disease. Never give up hope. Place your trust in the highest power. Rely upon the natural approach to resolve your health issues and, thus, put your body back into balance. The fact is the medicines of nature are powerful enough to restore human health.

This is a highly dangerous time. Unless information about what can be done is disseminated, lives will be lost. Unless all the data is made available, the human race itself could face dire consequences, perhaps a precipitous extinction.

There may be attempts to ban this book or, at the very least, interfere with its sale. Whoever does so only harms the general public. The fact is the contents of this book are based not upon folklore but rather modern science. This is why it is such a threat. The conclusions of this book, that the epidemics, even pandemics, can be cured, threaten vested interests which, apparently, stand to gain from human misery.

For tens of thousands of years natural medicines have be used to prevent and cure disease. Such information is in dire ne today. The ancients knew how to reverse disease. Today, tl information should be made common knowledge. Yet, ancie lore is insufficient. There must be proof from modern science. F wild spices and pungent herbs a plethora of scientific resear supports their use. The fact is, currently, there are a grea number of articles published yearly on the value of natui compounds than drugs. Thousands of scientific articles and boo are published every month, proving that various natui substances offer curative powers. Thus, the research on natu substances as successful medicines dwarfs that produc regarding synthetics.

I have predicted for several years that the world would sufi an international epidemic, sickening and killing hundreds thousands and even potentially millions of people. Now suck scenario is developing. It may strike, or if humanity establish the correct approach, it could be halted. Yet, such pandemics ha existed previously, not merely in ancient times but also in t recent past. Consider the decimation of Africa from AIDS a AIDS-like infections: hundreds of thousands die yearly. T cause is at least partly contaminated vaccines. Consider also t hepatitis C pandemic, which kills tens of thousands yearly.

Bizarre sex and AIDS

There have already developed pandemics, for instance, AIL This is largely a disease of the sexually deranged, that is it spread by unnatural sexual practices, particularly sex among me Infected men and women readily spread among natural partne Thus, the spread is out of control.

Evidence that AIDS is a bioweapon is lacking. What is certa is that, originally, its spread occurred through male-to-male se Many people blame monkeys. The habit of certain cent

African tribes of eating bush meat has been blamed. This certainly plays a role in the spread of disease. However, compared to sexual transmission it is a relatively minor one. Thus the main cause is the spread of germs directly through sexual encounters. Sexual promiscuity is the major factor in the spread of AIDS, and it is a significant factor in the spread of certain kinds of hepatitis, including hepatitis C. The spread of both of these diseases is directly tied to anal sex, which is practiced prolifically in homosexuals. The consequences of such practice are dire: the direct spread into the blood of immune-suppressive and organ-damaging germs, including various highly destructive viruses.

Anal sex isn't even sex. Physiologically, the rectum is poorly suited to receive the penis. Homosexuals must understand that this is highly damaging to their bodies. The blunt force of this organ traumatizes the rectal wall, causing bleeding. What's more, anatomically, in contrast to the vagina the fit is poor. While the vagina accommodates the penis, the rectum fails to do so. Thus, the hardened penis jams against an unforgiving rectal wall, ultimately ripping it. This leads to the seepage of rectal contents—human feces—as well as semen, into the blood. The results are diabolical: systemic immune, as well as internal organ, decimation. Semen itself is highly immune suppressive, and if it enters directly into the bloodstream, highly toxic reactions result. Even within men semen, if retained excessively, that is for prolonged periods, can be reactive.

God made the human being to be sexually active, that is, within the appropriate limits. Purposely avoiding the sex act, that is a celibate-like existence, leads to disease. The body must deal with the retained semen, which it regards as toxic. Imagine the toxicity of foreign semen is injected from one man to another. The results are catastrophic. Women have a protective apparatus: the thick-walled vagina. What's more, the vaginal tract contains secretions which limit or prevent any semen-induced toxicity. The rectur has no such protections. Thus, the persistent injection of seme into the rectum leads to a host of diseases, all due to the systemati destruction of the immune system. This may ultimately result i AIDS or similar potentially fatal infections.

Certain individuals commit bizarre acts. They have sex wit animals. The animals harbor a wide range of aggressiv pathogens. These pathogens readily enter the human body, that i through the rectum or urethra. Once there they mutate, developin into human pathogens. This ultimately results in chronic diseas such as kidney stones, chronic nephritis, cystitis, urethritis, coliti Crohn's disease, ulcerative colitis, and even AIDS.

The concept that AIDS has been inflicted upon the human rac by the 'government' or as a population control device is unfounde This is a kind of propaganda, perpetrated largely by the so-calle gay community. This is far from an attempt to "bash" a group c people. Nor is it an attempt to incite anger, hate, or retaliation. It i merely to set the record straight regarding the cause of huma epidemics. The fact is AIDS is most likely a mutation of variou animal pathogens contracted by freakish sexual practices, wher humans have sex with animals such as dogs, sheep, etc. Certainl such sexual interactions lead to infection within the human organ: Then, if such humans have sex with other humans, the cycle c transmission is perpetuated. Eventually, the pathogen develor sufficient power to not only infect but also potentially kill its hos This is the most likely origin for AIDS.

There is no medical treatment for AIDS or other chroni sexually transmitted diseases. Nor is there a medical cure fc SARS. This is the dilemma of modern medicine. Often, the caus of disease is unknown. This makes it exceptionally difficult t discover or create a cure. This is true of a number of infectiou diseases: the precise cause remains unknown. Or, there is only partial understanding of the cause. Lyme disease is an exceller xample. Once thought to be due to a specific bacteria, that is the pirochete, *Borrelia burgdorfi*, now it is known that a number of acteria and perhaps even viruses may be responsible. The oncept that it is polymicrobial, that is that multiple organisms re involved, makes sense. What's more, this has been confirmed y modern science.

When a tick attacks a person, it injects its saliva and perhaps lood into its victim. It also secretes its feces. Surely, these ecretions contain hundreds, even thousands, of pathogens. Vhat's more, many such pathogens originate from rodents, which cks feed on. Thus, much of the cause of this syndrome remains lusive. The fact is there are a number of germs deposited by ticks hich are unknown to science. This is why to a large degree accines and antibiotics are failing. They are designed only to kill ertain organisms, while the unknown organisms persist. The fact there will never be a successful vaccine against this disease. yme remains incurable, that is from a medical point of view.

Regarding natural medicines this is far from the case, that is ere are potential cures. A wide range of natural substances boost nmunity, aiding in the fight against this disease. A Polish study etermined that of some 38 herbs only one dramatically boosted nmune powers: wild oregano. It was this herb alone which ignificantly raised interferon levels, a marker indicating a direct nmune-boosting action. High interferon levels are a sign of nproved white blood cell function. This means that a wild regano supplement would serve as the ideal daily immune tonic, ne proven to boost immunity. Thus, the crude herb (i.e. the JregaMax original wild herbal formula) is a mainstay in the eatment of this disease. The latter is the maximum strength wild erb in a capsule. The extract, that is the oil, would also prove ivaluable. Its main function is to kill the pathogen(s).

Scientists are unaware of the mechanism behind most diseases. Vhen they develop a treatment, they often fail to account for

the complexity of such diseases. Thus, such treatments ar
usually doomed to failure. The antibiotics used to treat Lym
disease are an excellent example. The drug kills the bacter
which causes Lyme but fails to treat the viruses and parasit
which are also a part of the infection. Recently, it has bee
proven that ticks inject a wide range of germs. This is wh
despite such a treatment the majority of Lyme patients suffer onl
a partial cure, often outright relapses.

The single infection cause of disease is passé. Instead, th
majority of diseases are now being regarded as due to multip
infections. Take food poisoning as an example. Is it reasonable t
presume that when food is contaminated, for instance, by sept
water, as occurs in the tropics, the Middle East, or Mexico, that
person only develops one infection? When a person eats a foo
which is contaminated by raw sewage, is there only a single ger
contracted? The fact is there are thousands of types of germs i
infected water or sewage. If that water is consumed on food o
directly, the victim will likely develop a number of infection
Thus, the treatment with drugs which only target a single ger
may prove relatively useless. Consider gum infections. There ar
thousands of germs living in the mouth as well as on the gum
Would antibiotics, geared to kill single germs, truly be of value
Of course not. In fact they may usually aggravate the infectio
The same is true of urinary tract infections. Multiple germs ar
almost always involved. Treating such conditions with antibiotic
poses another problem: the creation of fungal infections. Th
urinary tract is lined with protective bacteria, which are norm
residents. Such bacteria act as a barrier, preventing th
overgrowth of certain pathogens, notably the yeast Candid
albicans. If antibiotics kill these protective bacteria, the Candid
overgrows, causing chronic infection. Candida is a viciou
pathogen. If it is allowed to gain a foothold, it can cause a wid
range of disorders. Symptoms of candida infestation includ

hronic headaches, sinus problems, spastic stomach, gas, loating, heartburn, spastic colon, fatigue, poor concentration, epression, anxiety, skin disorders, and allergies. Diseases ssociated with candida infection include irritable bowel yndrome, ulcerative colitis, esophagitis, Crohn's disease, hronic fatigue syndrome, chronic sinusitis, chronic bronchitis, sthma, lupus, kidney infections, bladder infections, prostate isorders, and arthritis.

The impact of emerging diseases is being minimized. People re dying, well before their time, and little if anything is done bout it. Preventive measures to help the public are virtually nknown, that is regarding emerging pandemics. The fact is such iseases are creating global havoc and have the potential for ausing great damage, physically and economically. In early 003 SARS had essentially shut down the Orient, causing vast uman and financial devastation. Beijing is at the center of a lobal attempt to curb the spread of this disease. In May 2003, iis massive city was cut off from the rest of the world, virtually ll its public and international activities coming to a halt. All was ue to a mere virus or, more likely, several viruses. The capital 'as so overloaded with new SARS cases that many hospitals ecame epicenters of the infection. "Due to the shortage of beds t designated hospitals", said Wang, Chief Medical Officer for ie region, "not all suspected cases could be hospitalized in a mely manner." What's more, as of May 1st some 10,000 people 1 Beijing had become quarantined, an incredible fact for such a iodernized city, fully overwhelming medical and social ystems. How will such a system handle, for instance, 100,000 r a million quarantined?

A cure is needed for SARS. In China and Hong Kong there is tter mayhem. Thus, the only hope for this region is to discover a ure. There is no way to contain it. It must be halted by killing the irus safely, that is without damaging or killing the patient.

The point is people are dying unnecessarily. There are number of preventive and even curative measures which, if the became known, would save lives. The fact that this has failed occur is largely due to a single issue: the machinations of the medical monopoly, which seeks to obstruct the dissemination of certain information. If such information fails to meet its agend then it is restricted, in fact, obstructed. Laws are establish prevent access and/or claims. For instance, there might be an her or food which blocks the development of, or even reverse cancer. Yet, no such statement can be made. Even if the claim are utterly true, they cannot be readily made, that is without ri of prosecution. This is an enormous impediment to the dissemination of correct information, so that effective cures ca become known.

Even if research is done proving an effect, often, claims are sti restricted, that is on the basis of so-called scientific agreement. other words, the claims can only be made if the existing scientif community agrees to their legitimacy. Or, they can be made on after the government, that is government-paid scientists, agre Yet, this is the case, even though such scientists often hav financial or social ties directly to the medical monopolies. In oth words, these scientists have an interest in minimizing or denyin the value of natural cures. Thus, under such a system the averag individual suffers, since legitimate information is withheld, in fac repressed.

The natural medicines, which are God-given, are impossible disprove. When a person eats an orange, he/she is consuming medicine, which keeps the arteries and veins healthy. When a perso takes oil of wild oregano, he/she is consuming a natural germicid which kills whatever is attacking the body, potentially saving th individual's life. If diarrhea strikes, unprocessed honey can be take which halts this symptom. These are not man-made. What right d humans have to "regulate", in fact, deny, them?

Today, people are dying from a wide range of infectious diseases, virtually all of them preventable. This means that if the appropriate natural medicines were popularized thousands of lives would be saved: daily. Since all else has failed in the treatment of various aggressive epidemics—AIDS, SARS, hepatitis C, Lyme, and similar debacles—certain natural compounds, which are truly effective, must be endorsed. Because such cures are repressed people continue to suffer, dying miserable deaths, all due to preventable, as well as curable, infections. Infected by a wide range of germs for which there are no medical cures, patients die in utter agony as doctors stand by helplessly. The fact is the majority of these lives could be saved: all through using natural substances.

Modern epidemics have barely begun. The worst will soon surface. Now is the time to ensure that herbal medicines, which are proven to kill viruses, are popularized. Oregacyn is highly antiviral. Studies at Microbiotest Labs have shown that this extract of wild spices completely obliterates the human coronavirus, killing all traces within 20 minutes. Other studies demonstrate the same action against cold sore, hepatitis, and flu viruses. Incredibly, in one study the viral counts in human blood were reduced from 5,000,000 to 450, a 13,000% reduction. The Oreganol P73 (oil of wild oregano) was also effective, killing 99.9% of the viruses. The Oregacyn is more powerful, because it is the state-of-the-art technology in concentrating the power of spice oils. Plus, it contains primarily three synergistic spice oils: wild cumin, sage, and oregano. It is, essentially, an antibiotic-like substance. In fact, it is more than this, because unlike antibiotics, which only kill bacteria, Oregacyn destroys the full range of germs: bacteria, viruses, molds, yeasts, and parasites.

It is time to educate people about the powers of natural medicine. This is the last chance people will have. If influenza, SARS, West Nile, or the bird flu develop into full-fledged pandemics, as appears to be the case, it will be too late. What is

certain is that these are far from eradicated: rather, they ar
looming, ready to strike at any moment.

By making this information known, thousands, perhap
millions, of lives can be saved. Much human misery can b
prevented. Billions of dollars can be saved. The infrastructure i
incapable of withstanding thousands of sick people, let alon
millions. All will utterly break down. The cure must be found a
well as popularized. This is in order to prevent wholesale deat
and devastation. It is in order that lives will be saved.

High quality natural medicines are risk-free. It is the man
made medicines which are causing virtually all the damage an
death. What is the harm of, for instance, trying a truly natura
medicine such as raw wild honey, apple cider vinegar, or oil o
oregano? A mere week's dosage of acetaminophen can caus
permanent liver damage. Thus, compared to such a harsh effec
there is no danger in the natural. Yet, for any major illness i
there a proper medical cure instead? Are the hospitals able t
cope? Does medicine have the answer? These are critica
questions, because the fact is in medicine herbal therapies ar
largely neglected, especially in medical establishments. Plus
they are repressed. Even if they are scientifically proven, the
are rarely if ever endorsed. Rather, a degree of hostility i
represented towards them. Such an attitude is ludicrous. What'
more, if people attempt all manner of herbal/natural medicines
what harm will be incurred? As long as a person sees his/he
doctor for any serious illness, there should merely be suppor
for any other non-toxic therapy attempted. The fact is with rar
exceptions there is no evidence that herbal medicines cause an
harm. The point is if it is safe and can do no harm and if ther
is a reasonable scientific basis, people should be allowed to tak
advantage of it. That is the ideal attitude in such a dire crisis
which threatens the very existence of human civilization. I
other words, in this instance human beings need all the hel

hey can get. No attempt must be made to restrict access to
potentially valuable substances.

The medical profession has proven incapable of curing
disease. There is no cure for heart disease, diabetes, high blood
pressure, or cancer. There is no cure even for the common cold.
Thus, how could one be found for SARS, AIDS, hepatitis C,
Lyme, West Nile, bird flu, or similar 'new' diseases? If after over
50 years of research and untold billions of dollars spent, no cure
can be found regarding, for instance, cancer or heart disease,
then, certainly, it is illogical to believe that a cure will be
discovered for emerging infections, which are ravaging
humanity: AIDS, West Nile virus, hepatitis, sepsis, Lyme, and
SARS. Thus, it is necessary to search in the natural medicine
kingdom for cures. The fact is this is where all cures are found.
Regarding modern plagues there is no hope for a medical cure.
Only natural substances can do so.

The challenge in medicine is that, usually, no one knows the
true causes. Unless the cause is known precisely, cures are
impossible to achieve. Thus, initial effort must be to determine
the cause. In other words, a precise diagnosis must be made.

With infection this may prove difficult. Yet, in a general way
the correct treatment can be applied. All that must be realized is
that the body is infected. Then, the immune system must be
bolstered. What's more, noxious germs must be killed. Once
such germs are killed the immune system is relieved of its
burden and good health will return. This is because natural
compounds are capable of killing a wide range of germs. For
instance, spice oils, such as Oreganol P73, as well as the multiple
spice oil concentrate Oregacyn, which comes in an easy-to-take
capsule, have been shown to kill virtually every type of virus.
Thus, all that needs to be done is to determine if there is a viral
infection. The type of virus is usually irrelevant. This takes the
fear out of emerging diseases, that is to realize that there can be

available an outright cure: regardless of the germ. Yet, Oregacy
also kills bacteria, parasites, and fungi, that is it covers the entir
gamut of infectious crises.

Modern medicine has utterly failed in the treatment/cure c
infectious diseases. The fact is in many instances it ha
perpetuated such diseases. *JAMA* (*Journal of the America*
Medical Association), has clearly delineated this. According to th
Journal modern medicine has created its own array of infectiou
diseases, for instance, drug-resistant staph, strep, candida
pneumococcus, and enterococcus. A mere visit to a hospital ma
lead to the onset of such an infection. In other words, by touchin
contaminated surfaces and then touching themselves people ca
infect themselves with potentially lethal germs. The same occur
through inhalation: the air in hospitals is overcome wit
pathogens. Thus, the unsuspecting 'visitor' becomes contaminate
with disease-producing bacteria or other germs, which coul
ultimately precipitate sudden infection and even chronic illnes
Such man-made infections prove that modern medicine will neve
develop true cures against the gamut of infectious epidemic
rather, it causes such epidemics. The *Journal* further documents
dire fact: that in hospitals alone a minimum of 250,000 individual
die every year as a consequence of antibiotic therapy, agonizing i
sepsis: all due to drug therapy.

Vaccines also fail to cure. They too instigate diseases. A va
range of diseases have been directly associated with thes
injections. Vaccine-induced diseases include:

- fibromyalgia
- polymyositis
- chronic fatigue syndrome
- irritable bowel syndrome
- multiple sclerosis
- myasthenia gravis

- lupus
- AIDS
- asthma
- SIDS
- arthritis
- pericarditis

- heart disease
- attention deficit disorder
- seizure syndromes
- Parkinson's disease
- brain cancer
- lymphoma
- benign tumors
- muscular dystrophy
- meningitis
- phlebitis
- Lou Gehrig's disease (ALS)

- cardiomyopathy
- Type I diabetes
- autism
- Alzheimer's disease
- leukemia
- bone cancer
- stroke
- Guillain Barré syndrome
- encephalitis
- nephritis

Consider this, that is the degree of harm, socially, physically, emotionally, and financially, caused by such diseases. The lives of uncountable people are destroyed, and, thus, civilization suffers. Yet, much of this damage is directly due to vaccines, a true modern medical debacle. Incredibly, the very treatment that people have learned to trust as protective is, rather, destroying them.

Vaccines cost the American public billions of dollars. This is because of the diseases which they induce. Yet, there is seemingly no means for recourse. The government has created legislation to prevent people from suing the perpetrators of this fraud. The fact is the vaccine makers themselves are well aware of the toxicity of their wares. Yet, how legitimate is such legislation, when it was created with foreknowledge: maliciously with an intent to defraud? Is that anything except a violation of the most extreme degree: of an individual's civil rights?

In this modern world the risks are dire, that is for encountering life-threatening infections. Violent forms of the flu, SARS, AIDS, Ebola, Lyme, drug-resistant staph, hepatitis B, hepatitis C, meningitis, and West Nile have proven this. Hospitals are exceptionally dangerous, that is due to the spread of mutant germs. What is an individual to do? Without a thorough knowledge of natural cures, what other hope is there? Surely, thi is the only hope for the future of the human race, that is to rely o natural cures, the very cures created for the benefit of humankind Some might dispute this point. Yet, who made them? How di perfect medicines such as raw honey, wild oregano, wild sage wild rosemary, ginger, cumin, cinnamon, cloves, and simila potent cures, arise? All these have direct and predictable action against germs. All aid the body's healing response.

Who perfected the chemistry of such potent natura compounds, which are equally as effective if not more effectiv than drugs? Did they arise on their own? If so, how could the work so perfectly, so effectively, within the human body? The must have been created for human benefit. Is there any othe possible conclusion? Thus they are the manufacture of the might one: the all-powerful and merciful God.

It is a mercy that human beings have such medicines. Wha would we do without them?

Natural medicines, in fact, work. They are capable of outrigh curing disease. They do so without significant side effects, tha is without causing the body serious harm. The same can never b said of drugs, which not only fail to cure but also, in fact, caus diseases. What's more, drugs can kill. This is rarely if ever tru of natural compounds. A careful analysis of death records prove this. For instance, from 2000 to 2003 there was not a single cas of death from natural substances such as garlic, oil of oregan oil of rosemary, cloves, cinnamon, echinacea, goldensea flaxseed oil, primrose oil, B vitamin or vitamin C tablets, natura (non-iron) mineral supplements, or similar agents. Yet, durin this time there were over 500,000 deaths from drugs. Th consequences are obvious: drugs kill, while herbal and natura medicines save lives.

Incredibly, regarding natural products people often ar concerned about side effects. It is reasonable to be cautious, tha s to be certain of safety, before using a substance. Regarding uch substances, the consumer might ask, "Are there any side ffects?" or "Is there any serious interaction with drugs?" or "Can t cause any damage (i.e. to organs or cells)?" Yet, does that same erson show even the same concern regarding the toxicity of lrugs, not just prescription ones, but also non-prescription? Does uch a person even consider the negative interactions from ommon over-the-counter drugs such as aspirin, ibuprofen, cetaminophen, H-2 blockers, and/or antacids? The interactions of such drugs with other drugs or with the various natural ompounds of the cells and organs is vast. This is the nteraction/toxicity to be concerned about, not the insignificant nteractions that might occur from herbs. The fact is the vast najority of herbs prevent toxic reactions, rarely if ever causing hem. In particular, edible medicines, that is foods, herbs, and pices, which are part of the normal food chain, are free of serious ide effects. Rather, they improve overall health. Deaths rarely if ver occur from such substances. In contrast to drugs, food-based upplements, such as garlic, onion, oregano, sage, and rosemary xtracts, prevent cellular poisoning, never cause it. What's more, uch substances help reverse the toxicity caused by drugs, even protecting the cells from such damage.

In previous ages the word drug applied to natural compounds. n fact, this term derives from Arabic. The original concept was o derive medicines from nature, which was popularized during he seventh century by the Prophet Muhammad. It was he who nade it clear that rather simple natural substances, such as spices, aw vinegar, and raw honey, as well as certain fruit, were potent nedicines. An entire empire flourished due to his teachings. During this era the word drug meant a compounded herbal nedicine, natural extract, or herbal food. For nearly 50,000 years of human history drugs were primarily vegetable. In the Islamic Era, when the concept of the herbal drug was created, this term

meant freshly produced herb- and spice-based medicines of a
types as well as food-like medicines. Today, drugs are synthetic
that is man-made.

Toxicity: what are the risks?

People wonder if a substance with such a high degree of power i
safe. The components of Oregacyn are derived strictly from
edible substances: wild mountain-grown spices. Such substance
are non-toxic. Other than an occasional upset stomach, which ca
be expected from hot spices, no toxicity exists. Thus, even in high
doses there is no liver or kidney risk. Rather, the Oregacy
reverses toxicity. The fact is, it is the ideal antidote for poisoning
especially from exposure to toxic fumes and/or chemicals. If
person is suddenly poisoned, it is the Oregacyn which ca
reliably reverse it. This is because the components of thi
compound dramatically increase the levels of one of the body'
key antidotes: the enzyme glutathione peroxidase. Thus, th
Oregacyn, as well as the Oreganol, is utterly safe for critica
organs such as the liver and kidneys. Rather, they boost th
function of such organs. If such organs are diseased, th
Oregacyn, as well as Oreganol, may be safely taken. In fac
human tests have documented the fact that through spice o
therapy the function of these organs is enhanced. A number c
studies have shown that the regular intake of the oil, that is th
Oreganol P73, in fact heals the liver, causing a normalization c
liver enzymes. In one instance liver enzymes, which were highl
elevated, i.e. SGOT level of over 400, were normalized withi
several months (i.e. SGOT level of 21). These cases wer
carefully followed. Clearly, in every instance it was the Oreganc
which caused the normalization. However, there is one issue
toxicity to the naturally occurring bacteria. In high dose
Oregacyn and Oreganol may kill the lactobacilli, which ar
somewhat sensitive to aggressive spices. So, in this instance it i

deal to consume prodigious amounts of yogurt as well as take a
igh quality natural bacterial supplement. In Oregacyn and
Oreganol therapy I use a highly effective natural bacterial
upplement known as Health-Bac. This never requires
efrigeration and, therefore, is easy to travel with. I find it highly
ffective in preventing diarrheal diseases when travelling. Ideally,
ake a half teaspoon at night in a warm glass of water before
edtime.

To avoid upset stomach spice oils should not be taken on an
mpty stomach. When taking such oils, always, at least initially,
ake them with food or juice. Later, when the body adjusts to
hem, they may be tolerated on an empty stomach. Yet, usually,
hey fail to cause any such symptoms.

Yet, people eat spices regularly and never consider the
onsequences. No one would consider spices toxic, because
hey are a food. Oreganol and Oregacyn are merely concentrates
f such spices. Therefore, they are non-toxic. They are also safe
o take with medication. There is one significant side effect:
hey reduce the need for medication. The aforementioned are
uaranteed to be non-herbal, that is they are made strictly from
oods. Avoid cheap imitations, in fact, counterfeits, which are
ot made from edible spices and which, thus, could be toxic.
oxicity can often be detected by smell. If the oil has a 'tinny'
r chemical-like smell—if it lacks the robust aroma that would
e expected from an oregano-tainted pizza or spaghetti
auce—avoid it, that is do not take it internally. There are a
umber of relatively inexpensive oregano oil products available
nade from farm-raised oreganos (in reality, marjorams) and
ven non-oregano species. Do not take such oils internally. The
73 designation is helpful: this is a guarantee that the contents
re made strictly from edible wild spice—the pungent oregano
sed by Greeks and other ethnics. The description "100% wild
igh mountain oregano", Mediterranean source, is also a sign

of quality. Brands which contain only spice oregano includ
North American Herb & Spice, Vitamin Shoppe, and Vivitas.

It is awareness and knowledge which will save the huma
race. This is the answer to the creation of a safer and mor
productive future. America can lead the world in this effort, bu
only if the people join hands in the performance of good deeds.
Americans join hands to create a positive, productive world, on
free of all forms of tyranny, then there is a chance for this worl
There is an opportunity to eradicate epidemic diseases. There is
possibility of saving uncountable lives. A Quranic phrase say:
essentially, 'If a person saves the life of another, it is as if he/sh
has saved the life of the entire humankind.' Now it is time to ac
to make this world secure and gain the profound benefit of th
greatest of all deeds: preventing the untimely death an
devastation of the living beings of this Earth.

Herbs, spices, food extracts and similar natural 'drugs' ar
made by an all-powerful Designer. Some may claim that the
evolve, that is develop on their own. This is senseless. There is n
evidence for such a claim. Yet, there is little evidence of thi:
Rather, it appears that each natural substance has its own uniqu
design: its own special chemistry. The question is would such
unique status occur merely by accident, as in evolution, or throug
deliberate creation? The answer is a matter of belief, yet, upo
consideration the involvement of an active Force is difficult t
deny. If such a Force created these medicines, then, ideally, thi
force—this all powerful being—would also create their recipien
Take oil of oregano as an example. This hot spice oil is a poter
antiviral agent. It kills viruses on contact. When taken internally
it destroys viruses without harming human cells. Ribovirin is
synthetic antiviral agent. It also kills viruses, yet it may readily kil
human cells, causing permanent damage. Interferon is anothe
example. Modeled after the natural type of interferon found i
cells, the commercial type is synthetic, made through geneti

ngineering. It too may aid in the killing of viruses, but like other
rugs, interferon readily kills human cells, even causing organ
amage. Natural interferon fails to do so, while the genetically
ltered/synthetic type does. Thus, the conclusion is clear: the
roducts of nature are safe, while the products of man-made
ntervention pose serious risks. Consider the consequences of
aking wild spice extracts—the reversal of disease:

CASE HISTORY: This is the exact wording of an e-mail received in
response to a radio program:

"Thank God for Oreganol...my two children, ages three and five years
old, and I were sick for over two months on and off with pneumonia,
pleurisy, and sinus infections. I was coughing up green phlegm for over
a month. I felt I was dying. I took two drops under my tongue each
night, after two days I started to feel better. In 12 days my lungs
completely cleared up. I rubbed a couple of drops on my children's
chests at night before bedtime, and they healed as well. Now I use it
when I see symptoms of a cold or flu and it clears up in a couple of days.
It's wonderful!

Thank You

Fann

Bibliography

Antonio, G. 1986. *The Aids Cover-Up? The Real and Alarming Facts abo* *Aids.* San Francisco, Ignatius Press

"Are Pigs Carrying Flu Superbug?", <u>The Times</u>, February 20,2004.

Burnett, F.M. Influenza virus infections of the chick embryo by the amneot route. *Exploring Medical Science.* 18:353.

Burnett, F.M. Studies on the combination with influenza viruses in the chic embryo III. Reciprocal genetic interaction between two influenza view *Exploring Medical Science.* 30:469.

Benson, A.S. 1985. Control of Communicable Diseases in Man. Washingto D. C.: American Health Publishing Association.

Beveridye, W. 1978. *Influenza: The Last Great Plague.*

Bray, R.S. 1998. *Armies of Pestilence: The Effects of Pandemics on Histor* Cambridge: Lutterworth Press.

Bush, L.M. 1935. *Common Sense Health.* New York: Liveright Publishin Corporation.

Clark, H. 1993. *The Cure for all Cancers.* CA: New Century Press.

Crosby, L.A. 1918. *Epidemic and Peace.* Westport, CT.

Drexler, Madeline. 2002. *Secret Agents.* New York: Penguin Press.

Elhs, M.E. 1998. *Infectious Diseases of the Respiratory Tract.* London: Cambridge University Press.

Garrett, Laurie. 1995. *Betrayal of Trust: The Collapse of Global Public Health.* New York: Penguin Press.

Garrett, Laurie. 2000. *The Coming Plague: Newly Emerging Diseases in a World Out of Balance.* New York: Hyperion.

Hubbert, W.T. 1975. *Diseases transmitted From Animals to Man*. Springfield, IL: Charles C Thomas.

Irwin, Alexander and Joyce Miller. 2002. *Global AIDS: Myths and Facts, Tools for Fighting the AIDS Pandemic*. Cambridge, MA.: South End Press.

Jensen, L.B. 1945. *Microbiology of Meat*. Champaign, IL: The Garrard Press.

Kocatn, G. 1999. *Flu*. New York: Simon & Schuster.

Marriott, Edward. 2003. *Plague: A Story of Rivalry, Science, and the Scourge That Won't Go Away*. New York: Owl Books.

McNeill, W.H. 1976. *Plagues and People*. New York: Anchor Press.

Oldstone, M.B. 1998. *Viruses, Plagues, and History*. New York: Oxford University Press.

Regis, Ed. 2000. *The Biology of Doom : America's Secret Germ Warfare Project*. New York: Henry Holt and Company.

Rhodes, R. 1997. *Deadly Feasts*. New York: Simon & Schuster.

Smith, Geddes. 1941. *Plague on Us*. New York: The Commonwealth Fund.

Stanier, R.Y. 1986. *The Microbial World*. Englewood Cliffs, NJ: Prentice-Hall.

Weintraub, S. 1998. *The Parasite Menace*. Pleasant grove, Utah: Woodland Publishing Company.

White, D.O. and F.J. Fenn. 1994. *Medical Virology*.

Index